Beyond Cortisone

Of Related Interest

Beyond Cortisone: Herbal Alternatives for Inflammation

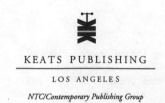

Martha Moore, A.H.G.

Foreword by Tieraona Low Dog, M.D., A.H.G.

KEATS PUBLISHING

LOS ANGELES

NTC/Contemporary Publishing Group

Published by Keats, a division of NTC/Contemporary Publishing Group, Inc.
4255 West Touhy Avenue, Lincolnwood, Illinois 60646-1975 U.S.A.

Library of Congress Cataloging-in-Publication Data

Moore, Martha, 1952-
    Beyond Cortisone: herbal alternatives for inflammation /
Martha Moore; foreword by Tieraona Low Dog.
        p. cm.
    Includes bibliographical references and index.
    ISBN 0-87983-837-X
1. Inflammation—Alternative treatment. 2. Herbs—Therapeutic
use. I. Title.
    RB131.M74 1998
    616'0473—dc21   98-55417
                                                    CIP

Printed and bound in the United States of America

International Standard Book Number: 0-87983-837-X
10 9 8 7 6 5 4 3 2 1

Contents

Foreword

It was a great pleasure for me to read the original manuscript of this book by Martha Moore. The conditions listed in this book are extremely common with millions of Americans suffering from arthritis, asthma, eczema and autoimmune disorders. The common approach is the use of pharmaceutical anti-inflammatories such as aspirin, ibuprofen, etc. and the much more powerful corticosteroids. These not only possess serious side effects such as gastric irritation, peptic ulcer disease, excessive bleeding, osteoporosis and immuno-suppression, but do not address the underlying disordered state of the body. Many chronic health complaints require an adjustment in lifestyle, diet and a common sense approach to alleviating symptoms while enhancing overall health.

Herbalists, in general, view illness within the context of the whole person and then choose herbs which support the specfic organ systems which are considered to be under stress. Most Western-trained herbalists believe that the body is a self-healing organism and that herbs should be chosen to support wellness and not simply to relieve symptoms. The body, mind and spirit are seen as indivisible and whole. The body is constantly applying a self-corrective force to maintain a delicate homeostatic balance in spite of illness, environmental pressures, poor diet, emotional stressors and life in general. Thus, herbalists choose remedies which can help the body maintain homeostasis, and therapy is directed at strengthening the individual's weakened areas with emphasis often being placed upon support of the adrenal and nervous systems.

Scientific research is currently available which validates the traditional uses of many of our ancient herbal medicines. A tremendous amount of money is being spent in Germany, France, Italy and numerous other countries in the pursuit of new knowledge about the medicinal uses of plants. Science is opening the door to a new, broader pharmacopoeia which encompasses both the pharmaceutical and botanical worlds.

The use of phytomedicine in today's world is as important to our well-being as it ever has been. The plants enhance our lives in so many ways. Who has not paused to take in the aroma of a rose and wonder at its beauty or experienced the healing which occurs during a walk through the woods or a field of wildflowers? Humankind has co-existed with the plant kingdom since our earliest days on the planet. We have evolved side by side. It is our responsibility to ensure the continued existence of all life, but especially the plants which provide us our very breath of life. Phytotherapy is a system of medicine which does not harm the environment (if harvesting/collection is done ethically), is available to all peoples throughout the world, is generally safer and, for the most part, far less expensive then most industrialized drugs. If we are going to achieve health care for all the 21st century, Western medicine must attempt to fulfill the recommendations set by the World Health Organization which clearly state that traditional medicines and practices need to be incorporated into the health care systems of every country. There is much to be gained and little to be lost with the incorporation of herbalism into mainstream medicine.

Ms. Moore skillfully weaves the biochemical and physiological role of inflammation in the body with its relationship to disease. Her approach to these disorders using herbs, diet and nutritional supplements is one which nourishes the body while reducing the harmful effects of inflammatory mediators. While symptoms are alleviated, a deeper healing is allowed to take place, which over time allows the body to regain wellness. Martha Moore easily integrates the best of historical folk medicine with up-to-date scientific research.

I am always thrilled that those who are seeking health have at their hands good, reliable literature. Anyone who is on this path of health will find this book to be an extremely valuable guide for addressing various inflammatory-related health problems. It can greatly benefit both individuals seeking to improve health and health care practitioners who wish to gain greater insight into a holistic model of medicine. It is with great pleasure that I highly recommend *Beyond Cortisone* to everyone who wants to address inflammation naturally.

Tieraona Low Dog, M.D., A.H.G.

Acknowledgments

Although the wisdom of many people has contributed to this book, I would like to express immense gratitude to all my herbal teachers including Tieraona Low Dog, M.D., Peter Holmes, L. Ac., Gary Smith, Michael Moore, Francis Brinker, N.D. and William Mitchell, N.D., who have been guides into the sacred gardens of medicinal plants, and to the plants themselves, who have been my teachers, healers and guides.

Moreover, I would like to dedicate this book to my parents, especially my mother for her tireless support and encouragement during this journey.

May the information in this book benefit those in need and help ease their suffering.

Introduction

Inflammation is a key feature in many diseases. Millions of people suffer from chronic inflammatory disorders such as asthma, autoimmune diseases (rheumatoid arthritis, multiple sclerosis, systemic lupus erythematosus), eczema, hayfever and allergies, inflammatory bowel disease (Crohn's disease, ulcerative colitis) and migraine headaches. Inflammation is a natural response, and can be beneficial for health. However, when inflammation is excessive or overactive it can damage healthy tissues and even contribute to the development of chronic inflammatory diseases and autoimmune diseases. Herbal anti-inflammatories and other natural approaches can help the body mediate inflammation and restore inflammatory balance. Medical doctors treat inflammation with anti-inflammatory drugs like NSAIDs (nonsteroidal anti-inflammatory drugs) and steroids that have adverse side effects, but the good news is that there are effective natural alternatives.

When inflammation causes chronic pain and swelling, it makes sense to modify it by approaches that do not cause additional problems. That is why herbal anti-inflammatories are often preferred to many of the pharmaceutical anti-inflammato-

1

ries. A range of safe anti-inflammatory herbs is available that treats inflammatory problems in a more gentle manner. Instead of attempting to eradicate inflammation it can be resolved in a holistic manner, thereby bringing the body back into balance. The use of herbal anti-inflammatories and nutritional supplements along with dietary and lifestyle changes offer us this potential.

What Is Inflammation?

Inflammation, or "in flame," is the body's reaction to tissue damage, foreign invasion or both. Although it is often viewed as undesirable because the effects can be unpleasant and cause discomfort, the process is optimally a normal and beneficial response to daily physical and environmental stressors. Without the inflammatory process, injuries would not heal and minor infections could become life-threatening. Inflammation is an important part of the body's immune response and can be activated or amplified by it. Equipped with elaborate defenses, the immune system fends off invaders, removes damaged or dead cells and maintains homeostasis. Inflammation may, however, develop at times and at sites with an intensity that is harmful, and the weapons intended to destroy invading elements or noxious stimuli may turn against the body itself. In these cases, the body fails to remove the noxious stimuli and becomes burdened with futile inflammatory reactions that produce debilitating effects and chronic disease. Any condition that ends in "—itis" theoretically refers to an inflammatory process, either acute or chronic.

CAUSES OF INFLAMMATION

The causes of inflammation are many and may be due to:

◇ Physical damage (trauma, wounds, burns, sunburns and radiation)
◇ Chemical substances
◇ Microorganisms (bacteria, viruses and parasites)
◇ Ischemia or death of tissues from lack of oxygen
◇ Foreign particles
◇ All types of immune-system reactions, including autoimmune conditions and hypersensitivity reactions, e.g., inappropriate or excessive immune reaction that damages the tissues.

It is this last category, in particular, which is integral to many aspects of inflammation.

THE INFLAMMATORY RESPONSE

Although the causes of inflammation can be varied, the sequences of physiologic events that follow are virtually the same regardless of whether the tissue damage or injury occurs on the surface of the skin or inside the body. For example, tissue damage or activation of the immune system releases inflammatory chemicals or mediators into surrounding tissues. Although these chemicals have individualized roles, they all cause the blood vessels to dilate (causing increased blood flow to the area) and to become more permeable or leaky, so that components that would normally be retained within the blood vessels are allowed to leak out into the tissue spaces. Plus, they attract immune-system white blood cells to the area in a process called *chemotaxis*. Chemotaxis brings white blood cells such as neutrophils and then macrophages to the injury site and promotes phagocytosis (engulfing and digesting bacteria or damaged tissues). The neutrophils also release powerful free radicals to kill bacteria or pathogens that could be in the area.

Signs of Inflammation

Four physical signs, called the four cardinal signs, characterize inflammation. The Roman physician Cornelius Celsus described them nearly 2,000 years ago: redness (*rubor*), heat (*calor*), swelling (*tumor*), pain (*dolor*). The Greek physician Galen added "loss of function" to the list of principal features.

ACUTE VS. CHRONIC INFLAMMATION

Inflammation can be acute or chronic. In acute inflammation the response is short-lived, lasting only a few days with an end result of healing or complete resolution of the tissues to normal. Chronic inflammation refers to longer-lasting inflammation and can become ultimately degenerative. An inability to mount an acute response causing chronic inflammation can be the result of (1) something that continues to provoke the inflammatory response such as a persistent irritant or foreign substance, (2) an under-functioning or deficient immune system due to disease, chemicals, drugs, age, poor nutrition or high stress levels; or as seen in a majority of cases, (3) an overactive or hyperactive immune system, such as occurs in allergies, asthma and autoimmune diseases like rheumatoid arthritis and lupus.

Immunologic mechanisms are believed to play a significant role in chronic inflammation. According to Simon Mills, "[t]here is a growing body of research that suggests that several chronic inflammatory diseases, often by definition with an autoimmunological element, are linked to low-grade chronic infections in separate parts of the body, and that either a cross-sensitivity is being set up to certain pathogenic antigens, or some toxic factor is being introduced."[1]

For example, excessive levels of toxin-producing bacteria in conjunction with inadequate amounts of friendly or normal bacteria in the intestines can result in a condition called "toxic bowel" or intestinal dysbiosis. These toxic bowel constituents can enter into the bloodstream by a condition referred to as "leaky gut" or abnormal bowel permeability. Many factors can lead to gut damage, allowing leakage of substances normally excluded into the bloodstream. For instance, constant exposure to food allergens can lead to irritation and inflammation of the small intestine lining, causing it to become leaky. Inadequate production of stomach acid (HCL) or digestive enzymes can also lead to increased inflammation of the small bowel by preventing adequate breakdown of food particles. Other factors that create intestinal inflammation and lead to abnormal bowel permeability include excessive alcohol intake; prolonged use of NSAIDs or broad-spectrum antibiotics; chronic intestinal infections due to viruses, parasites, yeast or bacteria and maldigestion.

Any of these mechanisms can allow increased absorption of large dietary and bacterial molecules or toxins to pass into the bloodstream where the body perceives them as "nonself" substances. These substances are called antigens and can lead to an increased immune/inflammatory response and promote food allergies. The body responds to these substances by forming antibodies to bind them. An immune complex forms when an antibody binds with an antigen. Although immune complexes are usually destroyed by phagocytic cells, at times these circulating immune complexes are deposited in other tissues. If they are deposited in joint tissues, for example, then immune cells destroy not only the immune complex but also damage the surrounding joint tissue. Furthermore, antibodies formed against these antigens can cross-react with the body's own tissues, causing autoimmunity. There is considerable documentation linking bowel toxins and absorption into the body with many autoimmune, immune complex and chronic inflammatory diseases, including rheumatoid arthritis, inflammatory bowel disease, psoriasis, lupus and others.[2]

Undesirable Consequences of Chronic Inflammation

In the case of chronic or degenerative inflammatory diseases, the body's wound-healing process somehow goes out of control and produces counterproductive, damaging effects. Excessive inflammatory responses that cause chronic swelling and pain, if allowed to continue, can result in progressive damage to tissues and body organs.

Additionally, a chronically inflamed area can produce so much cellular activity that there are more chances for genetic mistakes to occur, which can lead to the evolution of cancer cells. This is why it is essential to get rid of excess, unproductive inflammation in the body. The body has a number of cyclic nucleotides, and one of them is GMP (guanosine monophosphate) which tells the cell nucleus to divide like crazy and hyperproliferate. The enzyme, guanylate cyclase, stimulates GMP, and inflammation stimulates guanylate cyclase. In other words, inflammation in a tissue releases inflammatory chemicals such as leukotrienes and also generates free radicals to kill any bacteria present. Free radicals and leukotrienes stimulate guanylate cyclase, which stimulates GMP. GMP causes increased cellular activity that can lead to genetic mistakes and cancer cells.

Generally, overstimulation and toxicity cause cellular mistakes. If one is constantly toxic, leading the body to constantly produce free radicals to attack invaders, those free radicals are also damaging healthy tissues and transforming DNA into abnormal forms.[3] The toxicity control systems in the body can become dysfunctional if there is overactive free radical oxidation. Thus, antioxidants play an important role in modifying inflammation and protecting against free radical damage.

Inflammation—Good and Bad

As we have seen, the effects of inflammation can be both beneficial and harmful. Inflammation is initially a defensive and protective function, as in the destruction of invading microorganisms. It is the first stage in the healing process. We could not survive without it. However, sometimes acute inflammatory responses are inappropriate, such as those which occur in hay fever (type I hypersensitivity reaction). In these types of reactions, the provoking environmental antigen or nonself molecule, e.g., pollen poses no real threat. A hyperactive immune system causes allergies that in turn cause inflammation and tissue damage. It shows up as allergic rhinitis or hay fever in the nasal passages; in the sinuses, as sinusitis; on the skin, as hives or eczema; in the intestines, as food-allergy diarrhea; in the brain, as migraines; in the lungs, as coughs or asthma. These allergic-type inflammatory responses can be life-threatening, as in asthma. Thus, it is important to work with the body in modifying these inappropriate responses.

The destruction of normal tissue and free radical production are other potentially harmful effects of inflammation. Inflammation represents a major source of free radicals, especially in chronic inflammatory processes. The inflammatory response activates phagocytes, especially neutrophils, that trigger the production and release of free radicals to destroy bacteria, viruses or toxic chemicals. Free radicals as such are a result of tissue damage. However, if not quenched or deactivated appropriately, they can perpetuate or keep the damage going. Unless properly held in check by antioxidant defenses, a snowball effect or cascade of free radical production ensues. When inflammation becomes excessive or prolonged, it injures normal cells. It is then considered pathological, counterproductive and harmful. Long-term irritation causes degeneration of the tissues and disease. In these instances it is not a useful or appropriate response and causes injurious side effects. Indeed, even though some inflammations, like fever, begin basically as a healing process, harm might ensue when the intensity is excessive. Clearly, differentiating between beneficial inflammation and injurious inflammation is important in herbal medicine.

THE CELLS INVOLVED

Although understanding the inflammatory process may seem tedious, the more we understand it, the better we can modify its counterproductive or negative aspects by using herbal and other natural approaches.

Cells involved in inflammation include the following:

B Cells and T Cells. These are white blood cells (leukocytes) that carry the major responsibility for our immune response, recognizing and coordinating attacks against invaders. In addition, suppressor T-cells have an inhibitory action. They suppress the activity of both T- and B-cells, and are vital for winding down and stopping the immune response. They help prevent uncontrolled or unnecessary continued immune activity and are presumed to be important in preventing autoimmune reactions.

The herbs licorice, reishi mushroom, astragalus and Chinese wolfberry have all been shown to stimulate T-suppressor cell activity.[4]

Neutrophils, Eosinophils and Basophils. These cells release powerful chemicals (inflammatory mediators) that kill foreign invaders directly. Neutrophils produce antibiotic-like chemicals and cause a widespread type of cell killing by releasing germ-killing oxidizing chemicals into the fluid outside of the cell. However, recent research indicates that prolonged and excessively vigorous neutrophil activity can cause normal tissues to become cancerous.[5] Eosinophils and basophils are involved in allergic conditions and secrete histamine and other inflammatory compounds.

Mast Cells. These cells guard the body and act as "sensitive sentinels" detecting foreign substances and initiating local inflammatory responses against them. They are commonly found in connective tissue, throughout the walls of the respiratory tract and the intestinal tract surface membranes waiting for some invader or "nonself" substance to enter tissues from the bloodstream. Mast cells release histamine and other chemicals important in the response to allergens. When an antigen binds to an antibody, the mast cell degranulates and spews out or releases many inflammatory chemicals such as histamine, serotonin, inflammatory prostaglandins, leukotrienes, thromboxanes and platelet-activating factor. Together these chemicals induce an inflammatory response typical of allergic reactions such as hay fever, asthma and eczema.

A number of herbs have been shown to decrease mast cell reactivity and secretion, including licorice, dong quai, turmeric, ginger, Chinese skullcap, green tea and schizandra.[6] Many of these herbs are rich in flavonoids (plant antioxidants) which decrease inflammation by desensitizing mast cells thereby preventing release of inflammatory chemicals.

Essentially, the immune system recognizes foreign substances and acts to destroy or immobilize them. It protects the body from a wide variety of foreign agents as well as from abnormal body cells when it operates effectively. When it fails, malfunctions or is disabled, diseases such as cancer, rheumatoid arthritis and asthma may result.

INFLAMMATORY CHEMICALS OR "MEDIATORS" INVOLVED

Although inflammation has many different causes, its signs and symptoms are all produced by chemicals called "chemical mediators." Mast cells, basophils, neutrophils, eosinophils and other cells are responsible for releasing the chemicals that cause inflammation. Some of the chemicals released from inflammatory cells include the following:

Histamine. This is the best-known chemical mediator that triggers inflammation and it is widely distributed throughout the body. It is commonly found in mast cells and triggers the typical hay fever symptoms we are all familiar with: itching, sneezing, hives, runny nose, swelling, heat and soreness. Antihistamines block this inflammatory response.

Herbs that inhibit the formation or activity of histamine include Chinese skullcap, ginkgo, hawthorn, feverfew, tylophora and reishi mushroom.[7] Chinese skullcap, ginkgo, feverfew and reishi mushroom block the release of histamine from cells; hawthorn blocks the enzyme that permits the formation of histamine; tylophora has been shown to reduce histamine activity, however, the exact mechanism is unknown. Quercetin, a bioflavonoid found in many herbs and foods, also inhibits mast cell degranulation. In addition, merely drinking substantial amounts of water can act as a natural antihistamine because when the body is dehydrated more histamine is produced. Vitamin C can also help decrease histamine levels.

Prostaglandins. These are hormone-like substances that regulate cell functions in every part of the body including inflammation.

12

Some prostaglandins intensify and increase the inflammatory response while other reduce it, acting as anti-inflammatories. While there are a number of different types of prostaglandins, generally only three impact the inflammatory response. Series 1 and 3 are anti-inflammatory, while series 2 is pro-inflammatory. Series 2 inflammatory prostaglandins are produced from a fatty acid called arachidonic acid, found in animal foods like red meat.

Nonsteroidal anti-inflammatory drugs (NSAIDs), such as aspirin and ibuprofen, inhibit prostaglandin formation by suppressing the activity of an enzyme called cyclo-oxygenase. Cyclo-oxygenase converts arachidonic acid into series-2 inflammatory prostaglandins. Cyclo-oxygenase can also be inhibited, preventing the formation of inflammatory series-2 prostaglandins, by willow, ginger, feverfew, meadowsweet and by garlic and onions. In addition, glucocorticoid hormones (steroids) secreted from the adrenal cortex (or given as a drug, e.g., prednisone) act to suppress inflammation by inhibiting the enzyme phospholipase, thereby curtailing the availability of arachidonic acid for prostaglandin production. Likewise, licorice, chamomile, bromelain, feverfew and possibly turmeric also curtail the availability of arachidonic acid for prostaglandin production by inhibiting the phospholipase pathway.[8] Prostaglandin production can also be affected directly by certain dietary fats, since prostaglandins are made from fatty acids. Prostaglandins and dietary manipulation will be discussed in more detail later.

Leukotrienes. These are extremely powerful inflammatory agents. They are also produced from arachidonic acid but by a different enzyme, lipoxygenase. They are found in almost every body tissue and are capable of inciting strong inflammatory responses. Leukotrienes are an important inflammatory cause of asthma and acute allergic responses. They are 1,000 times more potent than histamine and 500 times more potent than inflammatory prostaglandins. A higher than normal level of leukotrienes is found in the skin or mucosa of those suffering from eczema and psoriasis, inflammatory bowel disease and allergic rhinitis (hay fever). Botanicals that interfere with leukotriene formation by inhibiting lipoxygenase include onions, garlic, chaparral, ginger, *Boswellia serrata* (an Ayurvedic herb), Chinese skullcap, quercetin and other flavonoid-rich botanicals.[9] Reishi mushroom has also been shown to reduce leukotrienes.[10] Other herbs and diet modifications can also inhibit the formation of leukotrienes by interfering with arachidonic acid formation since leukotrienes are made from arachidonic acid.

It is also worth noting that most fast-food pizza crusts are bleached with lipoxygenase, which can increase leukotriene production resulting in increased allergy and asthma problems.

Kinins. These are formed in response to tissue damage, allergy or other inflammatory sequences and are directly involved in causing pain, dilation of blood vessels, increased capillary leakiness and prostaglandin formation. Bromelain, found in pineapple, blocks the production of kinin, thereby reducing swelling and pain during inflammation.

Fibrin. Clotting-system factors form fibrin during the final step of the clotting process. Fibrin's role in the inflammation process is to form a matrix which walls off the area, resulting in blockage of blood vessels and edema. Although blood clotting

14

is an important function in tissue damage, it is equally important to prevent coagulation when it is not needed because clots can plug up vessels that must stay open if cells are to receive oxygen and nutrients and also to prevent excessive edema and swelling. Proteolytic enzymes found in botanicals like bromelain (from pineapple) and turmeric cause an increase in the breakdown of fibrin and help decrease swelling. Garlic and omega-3 type oils which will be discussed later also promote the breakdown of fibrin.

Platelet-activating Factor (PAF). This factor affects a variety of cell types and causes (1) platelets to clump together or aggregate reducing blood flow, (2) bronchoconstriction as seen in asthma, (3) increased blood vessel permeability or leakiness and (4) chemotaxis or attraction of immune ells and the release of their inflammatory compounds such as histamine and serotonin.

Herbs that inhibit platelet aggregation or formation of PAF include ginkgo, garlic, onion, ginger, dong quai, bilberry, cloves, and turmeric.[11] Omega-3 oils and proteolytic enzymes also reduce platelet aggregation, thinning the blood like aspirin but without the negative side effects associated with aspirin.

Serotonin. This chemical plays a role in allergic responses such as food allergies, asthma and migraines. In asthma it acts as another bronchial constrictor, and its release from platelets is a mechanism believed to cause migraine headaches. Feverfew is believed to inhibit the release of serotonin.

Thromboxanes. These are prostaglandin derivatives often associated with inflammatory conditions. They are released by a number of cells, including lung macrophages. They cause blood vessels to clamp down or vasoconstrict and play a role in the bronchial constriction that occurs in asthma. They also induce platelet aggregation. Thromboxanes are formed from inflammatory prostaglandins, which are formed from arachidonic acid. Their formation is promoted by a high animal fat diet and is inhibited by diets high in onions, ginger and fatty cold-water fish (caught in the wild) such as salmon, mackerel, sardines and tuna.

Free Radicals. These are highly reactive unstable molecules with unpaired electrons which can scramble the structure of proteins, lipids and DNA. Neutrophils, in a process called "respiratory burst," release free radicals which can cause damage to the surrounding tissue and alter molecules like collagen and DNA.[12] Although free radicals are normal by-products of the inflammatory response, if allowed to accumulate they can have devastating effects on healthy cells. Inflammation is a major source of free radicals in the body, particularly in chronic disease processes. In addition, free radicals are also produced by external sources, such as overexposure to sunlight radiation, environmental pollution, pesticides and second-hand smoke. This can all add up to an overwhelming load of free radicals internally. The free radical theory of aging postulates that free radical damage is what contributes to aging and degenerative diseases. In fact, over 100 degenerative diseases are associated with free radical damage and include autoimmune diseases (including rheumatoid arthritis), contact dermatitis, inflammatory bowel disease and many others.[13] Herbs and foods to modify free radicals are discussed in the next section.

BUILT-IN INHIBITING AND MODIFYING FACTORS

As discussed previously, the inflammatory response can result in the destruction of surrounding healthy tissues. This danger is lessened, however, by some modulating and moderating factors which are responsible for the self-limiting character of most inflammatory reactions. The surrounding healthy tissues have their own arsenal of defenses to protect themselves. They release anti-inflammatory prostaglandins to neutralize the inflammatory prostaglandins, antioxidants to combat the free radicals, antichemotactic chemicals to signal the white blood cells to stop coming in, proteolytic (protein-digesting) enzymes to break down the lysosomal enzymes produced by the white blood cells and enzyme inhibitors which inactivate inflammatory mediators.[14] In addition, T-suppressor cells help inactivate the immune response. These anti-inflammatory factors may be regarded as parts of a system which balance the generators of inflammation. These counteractive, anti-inflammatory responses allow the body to fine-tune its inflammation response and keep it in balance.

Causes of Inflammation Dysfunction

The inflammatory response can become imbalanced by a number of factors including:

◇ The body's overreaction to damage, creating an excessive, counterproductive inflammatory response.
◇ Inadequate deactivation, inhibition or quenching of the inflammatory process.
◇ Increased sensitivity or excessive activation of the inflammatory response through chemicals or drugs present in the body.

Optimally, in responding to injury, the body uses only those behaviors in the inflammatory sequence that are necessary to prevent or halt the destruction of tissue. It is a delicate balance, limiting the inflammatory process to the destruction of bacteria or the removal of only those tissues that are damaged so that other healthy tissues are not destroyed unnecessarily.[15]

EXCESSIVE INFLAMMATORY RESPONSES: THE ROLE OF ESSENTIAL FATTY ACIDS

The body's overreaction to damage causing an excessive, counterproductive inflammatory response is influenced to a great degree by the ratio of pro- and anti-inflammatory prostaglandins present in the body. These ratios are significantly influenced by dietary factors. Prostaglandin metabolism can be manipulated by altering the type and balance of oils or fats consumed in the diet. The kinds of oils we take into our bodies are incorporated into the cell membranes of our tissues and influence our inflammatory responses and cellular functions. If inflammation is a problem for you it is important to understand that inflammatory processes such as pain and swelling can be increased or decreased by eating certain foods.

The basic goal is to (1) reduce arachidonic acid levels, since inflammatory prostaglandins, leukotrienes and thromboxanes are produced from arachidonic acid (found preformed in animal fats), and (2) increase the level of essential fatty acids such as omega-3 fats which are usually deficient in the normal American diet and which lead to the production of anti-inflammatory prostaglandins.

Although most fatty acids can be synthesized by the body, certain unsaturated fatty acids required by the body can't be produced by it and must be provided by the diet and so are called essential. There are two families of essential fatty acids: omega-6 and omega-3. Linoleic acid (LA) heads up the omega-6 family and alpha-linolenic acid (ALA) heads up the omega-3 family. LA and ALA are considered the only "true" essential fatty acids because it is these two that the body cannot manu-facture and so must receive from the diet. LA is found predomi-nantly in vegetable oils such as safflower, sunflower, sesame, peanut and corn. ALA is found predominatly in flaxseed oil and in smaller percentages in pumpkin seeds, walnuts, soybeans and dark green vegetables such as kale and chard. After we consume these essential fatty acids, our bodies go through a complex series of steps to convert LA or ALA into various prostaglandins primarily through the action of enzymes. Thus, essential fatty acids and properly functioning enzymes are necessary for forming prosta-glandins which are the hormone like substances that modulate many important actions in the body, including inflammation.

Although there are several different types of prostaglandins, generally only three affect the inflammatory process: series 1 and 3 are anti-inflammatory and series 2 are inflammatory. As shown on the simplified diagram on pages 22–23, the anti-inflammatory series 1 prostaglandins (PG1) are produced from the omega-6 fatty acid dihomogamma-linolenic acid (DGLA). The PG1 series reduces tissue inflammation, such as that found in arthritis, among other functions. Evening primrose, borage and black cur-rant oils all contain GLA, which is the precursor for DGLA. Thus, GLA helps to make these series 1 anti-inflammatory pros-taglandins. Unfortunately, however, GLA is also a potential pre-cursor for arachidonic acid which triggers inflammation. In other words, DGLA can be metabolized both ways: into PG1 and into arachidonic acid, so it may be wise to use GLA supplements with caution as discussed below.

The series 3 prostaglandins are also anti-inflammatory and are produced from eicosapentaenoic acid (EPA) which is derived

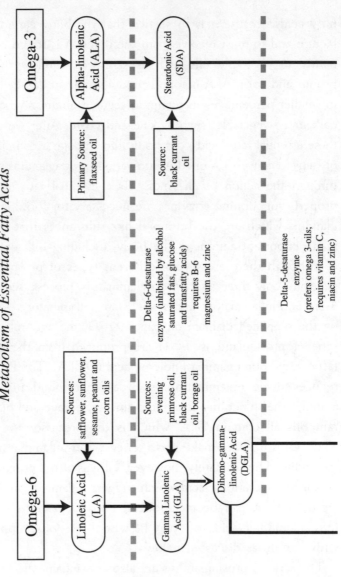

Metabolism of Essential Fatty Acids

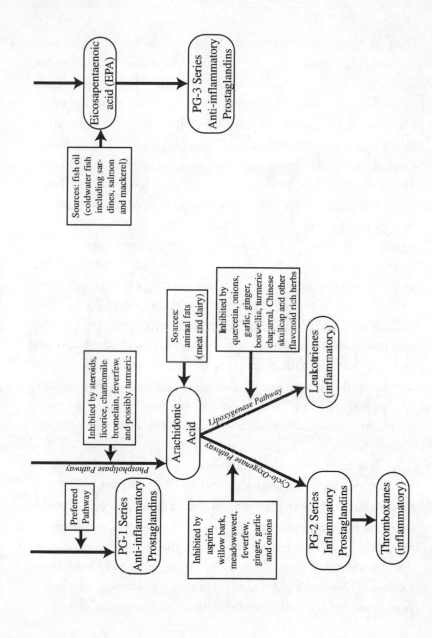

Eicosapentaenoic acid (EPA)

Sources: fish oil (coldwater fish including sardines, salmon and mackerel)

PG-3 Series Anti-inflammatory Prostaglandins

Inhibited by steroids, licorice, chamomile, bromelain, feverfew, and possibly turmeric

Sources: animal fats (meat and dairy)

Inhibited by quercetin, onions, garlic, ginger, boswellia, turmeric chaparral, Chinese skullcap and other flavonoid rich herbs

Arachidonic Acid

Leukotrienes (inflammatory)

Lipoxygenase Pathway

Cyclo-Oxygenase Pathway

Phospholipase Pathway

Preferred Pathway

PG-1 Series Anti-inflammatory Prostaglandins

Inhibited by aspirin, willow bark, meadowsweet, feverfew, ginger, garlic and onions

PG-2 Series Inflammatory Prostaglandins

Thromboxanes (inflammatory)

from ALA, the head omega-3 fatty acid found in flaxseed seed oil primarily. However, EPA can also be found preformed in cold-water fatty fish caught in the wild (not farm raised) such as mackerel, sardines, salmon and tuna; EPA is made by algae, plankton and seaweed consumed by these fish, so farm raised fish are not sources of EPA's. Thus, EPA can either be made from ALA by the body or consumed preformed in fish oils. These series-3 anti-inflammatory prostaglandins counterbalance the inflammatory prostaglandins and help return the body to normal functioning. The net effect of fish oil consumption is a significant reduction in inflammatory/allergic responses.

The pro-inflammatory series 2 prostaglandins, thromboxanes and leukotrienes are produced from the omega-6 fatty acid, arachidonic acid. Although arachidonic acid can be produced internally by the body from the omega-6 fatty acid DGLA, the enzyme (delta-5-desaturase) that performs this synthesis prefers omega-3 oils, so a large amount of arachidonic acid can be diet derived. Thus, some of the major agents of inflammation in the body (PG2's, thromboxanes and leukotrienes) are produced from arachidonic acid which is largely supplied by the diet.

Studies have shown that the more animal fats consumed in the diet, the more arachidonic acid in the cell membranes and blood and the higher the inflammatory chemical levels. On the other hand, a diet high in omega-3 oils, e.g., fatty cold-water fish and flaxseed oil results in a substantial reduction of arachidonic acid in cell membranes and a lower level of inflammatory mediators, plus a higher level of anti-inflammatory chemicals. Americans have greatly increased their consumption of arachidonic acid-rich animal fats in the last century, while reducing their consumption of fish and omega-3 oils. This may be one of the major causes for the increase in chronic inflammatory diseases that are now epidemic in our culture. In addition, alcohol consumption inhibits the amount of anti-inflammatory prostaglandins being produced, so this may also contribute to an excessive inflammatory response.[16]

There is evidence that a high intake of omega-6 polysaturated fats and a low intake of omega-3 fats increases the risks of developing inflammatory disorders such as rheumatoid arthritis and Crohn's disease. What's more, increased inflammation throughout the body can contribute to a wide range of conditions, including heart disease and stroke.[17] Diets high in omega-3 fatty acids can reduce arterial inflammation involved in coronary artery disease[18] and a study in the New England Journal of Medicine (1997), found that men with the highest levels of inflammation were three times as likely to have a heart attack and twice as likely to experience a stroke as men with the lowest levels.[19] The aspirin used in the study however irritates the stomach lining and can cause ulcers—omega-3 rich supplements, garlic, proteolytic enzymes (which will be discussed later) and other natural substances work extremely well in down-regulating the inflammation associated with these conditions without the side effects and complications of aspirin. Unfortunately, the American diet is high in omega-6 fats (LA) and very low in omega-3 oils (ALA and EPA). Most vegetable oils (safflower, sunflower, corn and sesame) have little or no omega-3 fats and are high in omega-6 oils. Other oils have a mixture of omega-3 to omega-6 in different percentages but the only common oil that contains a healthy ratio is flaxseed oil. In addition, although olive oil contains a small percentage of omega-6 oils, it is very high in oleic acid and therefore is not considered a contributor to arachidonic acid formation. Olive oil is high in monounsaturated fats which are slow to oxidize thereby lowering free radical reactions and is low in saturated fats, making it a good healthy oil to use for salad dressings and in cooking but it does not contain anti-inflammatory omega-3's. If we want our inflammatory process to function properly, we must eat diets with a high omega-3 to omega-6 ratio and avoid saturated fats (e.g. animal fats) as well as hydrogenated oils (e.g. margarine and shortening). Transfatty acids found in hydrogenated oils inhibit an enzyme critical to the production of anti-inflammatory prostaglandins and also cause leaky cell membranes disrupting cellular metabolism and permitting toxic substances to enter the cell.

As mentioned earlier, the process of transforming essential fatty acids into other forms that can be used by the body is accomplished mainly through the actions of enzymes. Unfortunately many of us have poorly functioning enzymes, such as delta-6-desaturase, which are necessary to convert dietary fatty acids into prostaglandins. Many physiological conditions inhibit delta-6 desaturase and reduce the body's ability to produce the counterbalancing anti-inflammatory prostaglandins. Delta-6-desaturase is inhibited by (1) the over consumption of sugar, (2) excessive dietary saturated fats, (3) release of adrenaline due to stress, (4) high alcohol consumption, (4) high blood cholesterol, (5) excessive transfatty acids, (6) zinc deficiency, and other factors.

For this reason, it may be wise to use dietary supplements and foods which are further down the metabolic pathway. Supplementation with evening primrose oil, black currant oil or borage oil (sources of omega-6 GLA) or fish oils (sources of omega-3 EPA) bypass the potentially weak enzyme. Experts believe, however, that for GLA supplementation to be effective, one must simultaneously restrict animal protein in the diet and supplement with omega-3 oils to help avoid any potential conversion into inflammatory prostaglandins.[20]

Although GLA supplements are quite popular, the research on GLA supplementation is controversial. Some studies have shown that long-term GLA can actually increase arachidonic acid levels and lower EPA (omega-3) levels, which is contrary to inflammatory treatment goals. Other studies have reported positive anti-inflammatory results.[21]

Supplementing with the omega-3 EPA fish oils also bypasses the potentially weak delta-6-desaturase enzyme. The studies in fish oil supplementation for rheumatoid arthritis have produced better anti-inflammatory and more consistent results than the studies with GLA supplementation.[22] Supplementation with 2 to 3 grams per day of omega-3 EPA (approximately 2 capsules of omega-3, three times a day with meals) is the recommended dosage. Concerns about fish oil supplementation include potential oxidation and rancidity. However, some high-quality sources are now available. (See Resources.)

In order to circumvent problems associated with fish oil and GLA supplementation, other practitioners believe that flaxseed oil is the best choice. Flaxseed oil is made up of approximately 50–58 percent of the omega-3 fatty acid (ALA), 14–16 percent of the omega-6 fatty acid (LA) and also contains omega-9 oils and others. However, flaxseed oil must rely on the body's ability to convert ALA to EPA by the potentially weak enzyme delta-6-desaturase.

William Mitchell, N.D., believes that balancing the fatty acid intake so that there are relatively more omega-3s is desirable in treating any condition that is inflammation-dependent and recommends flaxseed oil over other options. Mitchell believes this is especially true since omega-3 fatty acids are not precursors for the inflammatory prostaglandins as the omega-6 GLAs potentially are and are much less reactive in the whole hypersensitivity picture than omega-6 fatty acids.[23]

Even Hippocrates recommended flax (*Linum usitatissimum*) for inflammation, and the species name itself indicates that it was a "most useful" plant. However, for maximum effect, one study indicates that while supplementing the diet with flaxseed oil there should be a restriction of other vegetable oils, i.e., corn, safflower and other LA rich omega-6 oils in order to produce comparable effects as fish oil supplementation in lowering arachidonic acid and raising EPA levels.[24]

The recommended dosage for flaxseed oil is 1–2 tablespoons daily. Homemade salad dressings offer a great opportunity to add flaxseed oil to the diet. Add 6 Tbsp. of flaxseed oil to ½ cup of rice vinegar and combine with 2 Tbsp. of water, 2 cloves of minced garlic, some chopped onion, 2 tsp. dried mustard, ¼ tsp. salt and 4–5 Tbsp. of chopped fresh herbs, such as parsley, chives or cilantro. Combine all ingredients and blend completely. Make sure that you buy refrigerated flaxseed oil and look at the press and expiration dates to make sure it is fresh. Never use flaxseed oil or other unrefined highly unsaturated oils for cooking since they are easily oxidized when heated. They must be kept in the refrigerator, away from heat and light.

To recap, fish oils are not potential precursors for inflammatory prostaglandins like GLA and, unlike flaxseed oil, directly deliver EPA to the body and bypass the potentially weak enzyme needed for conversion of ALA to EPA. Although health care professionals have previously recommended flaxseed over fish oil as a source of omega-3 fats, the ability of manufacturers to now produce cost-effective, high-quality fish oil supplements enlarges your options. Further research in this area will hopefully clarify the clinical advantages or disadvantages among GLA, flaxseed oil and EPA-rich fish oil.

INADEQUATE QUENCHING OF INFLAMMATION: THE ROLE OF NUTRIENTS

Antioxidants. There are several different built-in mechanisms that limit the intensity and duration of the inflammatory response. In addition to the anti-inflammatory prostaglandins we have discussed, antioxidants can inhibit the production of pro-inflammatory chemicals and assist in controlling or quenching the inflammatory process. Antioxidants act as a counterbalance to the inflammatory process and help maintain homeostasis.

Carotenes are potent free radical quenchers and much more potent than vitamin E. One familiar example of a carotene is beta-carotene, which is found in carrots. Carotenes are also found in yams, pumpkins and dark leafy greens such as kale or chard. Herbs high in carotene include calendula, hawthorn and turmeric. The first two can be drunk as beverage teas, while turmeric can be added to meals as a spice.

Like carotenes, bioflavonoids exhibit a powerful ability to protect against free radical damage and help decrease allergic and inflammatory reactions. Bioflavonoids inhibit several chemical mediators including histamine, prostaglandins, leukotrienes and kinins and help stabilize the membranes of inflammatory cells that secrete inflammatory chemicals so they don't over-react.[25] Thus, bioflavonoids act as natural antihistamines and have a strong antiallergy action in many people.

Proanthocyanidins are another category of flavoniods found in many botanicals including hawthorn and most notably in pine bark and grape seeds. Research indicates that proanthocyanidins significantly decrease the inflammation and swelling induced by serotonin and prostaglandins.[26] Anthocyanidins are another type of flavonoid whose pigments create the red to purple and blue colors in blueberries, cherries, grapes, raspberries, bilberries and blackberries. Anthocyanidins and proanthocya-nidins both have profound anti-inflammatory effects and seem to have an affinity for connective tissue and collagen, promoting regeneration and stability of the connective tissues. Thus, they would be useful in many inflammatory conditions, particularly arthritis.

Quercetin is another flavonoid that functions as an antioxidant, quenching free radicals. Quercetin also reduces inflammation by blocking production and release of inflammatory agents. It is found in yellow onion, apples, kale, broccoli, russet potatoes, calendula, chamomile, hawthorn, gingko and numerous other pigmented foods and herbs. Available in a concentrated supplement form, quercetin is purported to be one of the most potent natural anticancer agents known.

Botanicals high in flavonoid anti-inflammatories include pineapple (contains bromelain as well as flavonoids), calendula, turmeric, chamomile, St. John's wort, ginkgo, bilberry, hawthorn, elder berry, linden, milk thistle and Chinese skullcap. It should be noted that some of these herbs have a particular affinity for different areas of the body. For example, St. John's wort has an affinity for the connective tissue such as tendons, joints and muscular tissues and also for nervous system tissues, whereas milk thistle has an affinity for the liver and has marked anti-inflammatory and liver protective effects. Milk thistle is believed to stabilize the liver cell membrane through its antioxidant activity. That is, it appears to restructure the outer cell membrane, stopping penetration of toxins into the cell's interior. Chamomile, on the other hand, has an affinity for inflammations of the stomach and bowels, such as IBD, colic and spastic colon.

Other flavonoid-rich extracts which are potent antioxidants and anti-inflammatories include curcumin and green tea.

A deficiency of these antioxidants/bioflavonoids in our diets can contribute to normally beneficial inflammatory processes going out of control, creating an excessive inflammatory response. As such, it is important to eat a variety of colorful or brightly pigmented foods and to supplement the diet with botanicals and nutrients rich in these components. The importance of antioxidants cannot be overstated in the treatment of inflammatory conditions.

Proteolytic enzymes. Another protective mechanism the body uses to keep the inflammatory response in check is the use of

31

proteolytic (protein-digesting) enzymes, and supplementing the diet with these enzymes can help mediate inflammation. Our bodies naturally produce these enzymes to digest food, to regulate metabolism and to regulate components of inflammation. Proteolytic enzymes (also called proteases) are one kind of pancreatic digestive enzyme. They support and accelerate the natural inflammatory process, assisting it from getting out of control. Specifically they have been shown to help: break down blood proteins that cause inflammation; remove "fibrin", which is the clotting substance that prolongs inflammation; clear up edema (reduce swelling) in inflammation areas; and counteract chronic, recurring inflammation. Proteolytic enzymes are often effective in the treatment of many acute and chronic inflammatory conditions. For instance, they have been shown to be useful in severe or chronic inflammatory conditions which are associated with increased levels of circulating immune complexes such as rheumatoid arthritis, lupus, scleroderma, ulcerative colitis, Crohn's disease and multiple sclerosis.[27] Proteolytic enzymes appear to safely lower serum levels of C-reactive protein which is a nonspecific marker in the blood for acute-phase responses to infectious agents, foreign substances and tissue damage. In other words, a C-reactive protein (CRP) analysis of the blood is a measure of the body's inflammation levels. In addition to reducing CRP levels in the body, these enzymes also improve blood flow and reduce the risk of blood clots, thereby improving circulatory health. Thus, these enzymes are another safe alternative to asprin or other blood thinners helpful in reducing heart disease but make sure you consult your health care professional before self medicating, reducing or changing any medications you may be on. It is important to remember that circulatory problems especially in the elderly may involve serious conditions. Thus, accurate medical diagnosis and proper monitoring by a health care professional is extremely important.[28]

Proteolytic enzymes are important, especially during the inflammation process, since they help the body to dispose of undesirable protein or wastes left over from tissue repair. These enzymes accelerate the "housecleaning" of injury waste matter, reducing inflammation time and accelerating the healing and repair process. Studies also show that proteolytic enzymes like papain (from papaya) and bromelain (from pineapple) effectively reduce pain and swelling in acute inflammations such as occur in sports injuries.[29] Furthermore, these enzymes are important for protein digestion and play a major role in keeping the small intestine free from bacteria, yeast, and protozoa. As such they would be helpful in avoiding intestinal dysbiosis and leaky gut syndrome. Using digestive enzymes helps break down foods into fundamental, well-absorbed nutrients and decreases the likelihood of immune responses to undigested food particles. In fact, studies show these enzymes to be effective in treating food allergies.[30] Moreover, proteolytic enzymes combined with flavonoids and vitamin C have demonstrated anti-inflammatory effects comparable to NSAIDs but without the side effects.[31] The normal dosage for bromelain is 400–600 milligrams, 3 times per day in between meals, unless it is being used as a digestive aid, then take with meals. As an alternative, juice ½ a pineapple along with approximately ¼-inch slice of fresh ginger root and drink daily to reduce pain and inflammation.

An effective enzyme combination supplement for reducing inflammation and pain would generally contain pancreatin (100 mg per tablet), bromelain (50 mg per tablet), papain (50 mg per tablet), amylase and lipase (10 mg each per tablet), trypsin and chymotrypsin (100 mg per tablet). Dosage is dependent on individual product quality and potency but generally, 5-10 tablets, 3-4 times per day on an empty stomach is recommended for anti-inflammatory effects. Alternatively, pancreatin (10X) can be taken alone: 350-700 mg 3 times per day in between meals (on an empty stomach) for anti-inflammatory effects or immediately before meals as a digestive aid.

Excessive Activation by Drugs/Chemicals

Many food additives (colorings, flavoring, preservatives and emulsifiers) and environmental toxins can either increase sensitivity to inflammatory reactions or can directly activate excessive inflammatory processes inappropriately. Research has shown that food and drug additives, such as artificial colorings, flavorings, chemical preservatives and emulsifiers, cause inflammatory problems, especially in those people suffering from asthma and eczema.[32] The coloring agents that cause the biggest problems are the yellow ones produced from tartrazine. These are commonly found in cheddar cheese, cheese puffs and candies. Other chemicals are added to improve taste, including MSG, aspartame and salicylates. Salicylates are known to trigger asthma and hives in sensitive people. Chemical preservatives can also create problems, especially nitrites, sulfites, benzoates and sorbic acid. Emulsifiers and stabilizers are also added to our foods to increase bulk or weight. Some of these, such as polysorbates and vegetable gums (e.g., carrageenan) increase sensitivity to inflammatory reactions and are associated with chronic inflammatory bowel disease in some people.

Restoring Inflammatory Balance

A high percentage of people who eat the typical American diet suffer some degree of inflammatory imbalance. The first step in restoring balance is to decrease inflammatory prostaglandins in the diet primarily by decreasing arachidonic acid rich animal fats and to increase the level of anti-inflammatory foods, supplements and herbs. It is also important to avoid chemicals that create excessive inflammatory stimulation. This would include decreasing exposure to sources of free radicals in the environment by avoiding excessive ultraviolet sunlight, eating pesticide-free organically grown foods with no chemical additives and avoiding contact with toxic household and industrial chemicals.

It takes consistency, time and commitment to change the essential fatty acid components in the body because it is not only the fatty acids in the blood and the cell membranes that are out of balance, but all of the body's fat stores. In a typical adult approximately 30 percent of the body weight is fat, so a man who weighs 180 lbs. is potentially carrying around 54 pounds of imbalanced fatty acids. Thus it would take a long time to correct the imbalance by diet alone. That is why, in addition to diet changes, supplementing the diet with herbs and nutrients, such as high-quality EPA supplements or balanced fatty acids like flaxseed oil, is recommended while at the same time cutting back on omega-6 vegetable oils and arachidonic acid-rich animal foods. This commitment to restoring inflammatory balance naturally is easier when you consider some of the serious problems associated with taking anti-inflammatory drugs.

ANTI-INFLAMMATORY DRUGS

More than 200 potential anti-inflammatory drugs, ranging from nonsteroidal anti-inflammatory drugs (NSAIDs) and corticosteroids to gold salts, methotrexate, and hydroxychloroquine, are prescribed by doctors, but all are known to produce side effects, many of which are very serious. Pharmaceutical corticosteroids, commonly called steroids, are occasionally needed for acute inflammation/immune suppression and can rapidly relieve the pain, swelling, and redness caused by inflammation. But these are powerful drugs that have serious side effects especially when taken for long periods of time. Side effects may include lowered resistance to infection, depression and other mental/emotional disturbances, high blood pressure, diabetes, cataracts, blurred vision, loss of muscle mass and strength, serious stomach problems such as peptic ulcers, thinning and weakening of the skin and osteoporosis.

The most common and popular inflammation relievers are NSAIDs, which include aspirin, acetaminophen (Tylenol), ibuprofen (Advil) and others. These can cause stomach bleeding and ulcers, gastrointestinal distress (heartburn, nausea, stomach pain, vomiting, diarrhea), headaches, dizziness and/or tinnitus. More serious complications can include kidney and liver damage. In addition, these drugs appear to accelerate osteoarthritis and promote increased joint destruction.[33]

Although it may take up to six to eight weeks, or in some cases up to several months, to notice the benefits of dietary change and nutritional and herbal supplements, these natural approaches, unlike pharmaceutical drugs, can be effective and are not accompanied by negative side effects when used correctly.

Herbal Approaches to Inflammation

Unlike allopathic medicine, herbalism, acupuncture, naturopathic medicine and other complementary modalities approach the healing of chronic illness as much more than a suppression of symptoms. Most complementary approaches work on the whole body, increasing vital energy, restoring metabolic balance and bringing increased tone to the organs. They increase the body's ability to deal with illness and inflammation. Utilizing a broad holistic approach, herbalism assists in resolving the condition while alleviating pain and discomfort. It is not aimed at simply alleviating symptoms; it also focuses on liver function, circulation and elimination, as well as quality of life. It is important to realize that although herbs play a central role in moderating inflammation, other approaches like acupuncture, nutritional supplemention, diet and meditation are also important in restoring internal balance.

Herbs can work with chronic inflammation in a variety of different ways. Most herbal anti-inflammatories act to slow, not halt, the inflammatory response. Completely stopping the inflammation impairs the body's ability to "take out the trash" or remove toxic debris. It is important to help the body remove wastes from injured tissue, not to stop the inflammatory process entirely as with pharmaceutical drugs. Herbs also nourish injured tissues, unlike pharmaceutical anti-inflammatories.

Herbally, the main approach is to modify the inflammatory process by stimulating anti-inflammatory functions and stimulating eliminative, circulatory and metabolic functions. Herbal formulas traditionally used for inflammation, in addition to direct anti-inflammatory herbs, include:

1. **Circulatory stimulants** (e.g. prickly ash, ginger, garlic, guaiacum)

2. **Diuretics** (e.g. celery seed, nettles, yarrow, yerba mansa, dandelion leaf)

3. **Mild laxatives** (e.g. dandelion root and yellow dock)

4. **Bitter herbs** to stimulate digestion and detoxify the liver (e.g. bogbean, barberry, dandelion root, gentian, wormwood, milk thistle).

5. **Lymphatics** to assist the tissue-cleansing activity of the lympathic system (e.g. cleavers, fenugreek, calendula, goldenseal, red root).

6. **Nervines** to calm, relieve anxiety and nourish nerve tissue (e.g. St. John's wort, lemon balm, passion flower, kava kava, chamomile, linden, skullcap) and **adaptogens** to help deal with chronic stress (e.g. siberian ginseng, ashwagandha, reishi).

7. **Alteratives,** herbs which gradually restore proper body function and increase vitality, are specifically indicated in chronic inflammatory conditions. Their mode of action is unclear, but many of them enhance the body's ability to eliminate waste, assist in

detoxification, stimulate digestion, enhance nutrition and probably have other less understood actions. (e.g. burdock, dandelion, red clover, nettles, guaiacum, bogbean and horsetail).

Dandelion has long been used for treating chronic diseases since it enhances digestion, assimilation, metabolism and elimination. Herbs such as horsetail and gotu kola which increase the repair and regeneration of connective tissue, are also helpful in inflammatory diseases like arthritis and lupus. Thus, many herbal anti-inflammatory remedies work by encouraging the inflammatory response in its task of cleansing, removing and repairing rather than merely suppressing it. Herbs have an important advantage over conventional drugs since herbs have a broader range of possible actions, particularly when taken in combination. They work synergistically to strengthen and assist the body in its healing processes in many different ways at the same time that they relieve symptoms.

Many herbalists believe that it is a mistake to simply inhibit the inflammatory response, particularly in acute inflammations, which usually are self-limiting anyway. If allowed to run its course or by merely supporting the body's efforts to speed recovery, an acute inflammation can perform its function of discharging the original disturbance and the body can return to a state of health. On the other hand, if the inflammatory response is self-perpetuating, inappropriate and counterproductive, it is important to directly address the symptoms in an attempt to break the cycle causing the damage or to neutralize the overactive response and offer relief from chronic pain. The goal in treating chronic inflammation is to bring back into balance an out-of-control, destructive mechanism.

Types of Herbal
Anti-Inflammatories

For the Latin names of the herbs discussed here and in subsequent chapters, check individual listings in the Concise Materia Medica, pp. 93–125. For herbs not listed in the Concise Materia Medica consult the Appendix at pp. 129–131 for a listing of latin names and plant parts used.

Herbal anti-inflammatories can be categorized into groups according to chemical constituents or the way in which they are thought to work. Although plants are complex entities with properties that cannot be simply reduced to a list of constituents, this chemical analysis is clinicially useful especially when put in relation to other facts such as clinical trials or empirical usage. Indeed, in many cases these scientific conclusions merely affirm traditional well known actions. It cannot be stressed enough that the action of any herb is always more than any specific chemical constituent or single mode of biochemical activity. In other words, the whole is more than the sum of its parts. With this holistic viewpoint in mind let us examine the different herbal anti-inflammatory groups.

SALICYLATE-CONTAINING HERBS

Many plants contain natural aspirin-like compounds called salicylates. Indeed, all the aspirin-type drugs were originally isolated from natural plant sources. It is interesting to note that the term aspirin comes from the old botanical name for meadowsweet—*Spiraea* (*aspirin*)—and that the term *salicylate* comes from the Latin botanical name for willow—*Salix*. The salicylate-containing herbs include meadowsweet, wintergreen, the bark of aspen and cottonwood, birch, black cohosh and willow, plus blackhaw and crampbark. Even though most willow and poplar barks contain phenolic glycosides such as salicin which are converted to salicylic acid in the intestinal tract and liver, the principal salicin-rich sources are *Salix purpurea* and *Salix fragilis*. These salicylate-containing herbs inhibit inflammatory prostaglandins and thus the proinflammatory process.

Salicylate-rich herbs need about six to ten hours of consistent doses to achieve a therapeutically adequate and steady blood level, however, so they are not very effective for acute inflammatory use. They reach optimal effectiveness only after three days. Thus, they don't tame a headache as quickly as aspirin, but they are extremely effective for chronic pain and inflammation such as chronic arthritic pain or chronic joint aches.

In addition, these herbs do not cause the same problems that aspirin can in the stomach. Unlike the acetylsalicylates in aspirin, which are broken down in the stomach and can irritate the stomach lining causing bleeding and ulcers, the salicylic precursors in these herbs are broken down in the intestines. These compounds are transformed to *saligenin* by intestinal microorganisms and then oxidized into salicylic acid in the liver and blood. Because these herbs are not metabolized the same way as aspirin, they are far gentler on stomach tissue.

Although salicylate side effects are unlikely since the salicylate precursors are not metabolized the same as aspirin, caution may be appropriate in those who have aspirin sensitivities. In addition, although Reye's syndrome has not been reported with the use of salicylate herbs they should not be used to lower fevers in children to avoid any possibility of Reye's syndrome.

STEROIDAL AND TRIPERPENOID SAPONIN-CONTAINING HERBS

Saponins are a type of plant glycoside that are divided into different classes, such as steroidal saponins and triterpenoid saponins. These two classes of saponins are similar in structure and activity, but we will look at them separately.

Steroidal Saponins. As with salicylates, steroids were also first isolated from plants, and there are several herbs that can be metabolized by the body into inflammatory-fighting steroid substances. Some contain steroid structures which are very close to the body's own natural anti-inflammatory hormone, cortisone, while others enhance the action of cortisone. Licorice, wild yam, yucca, sarsaparilla and fenugreek are examples of saponin-rich steroidal anti-inflammatory herbs.

Licorice contains the steroidal saponin, glycyrrhizin, which appears to produce anti-inflammatory effects by binding to steroidal receptors in the body. Moreover, it inhibits an enzyme in the liver which breaks down the body's own natural cortisone, keeping it available longer. Our own natural cortisone (corticosteroid) is a powerful anti-inflammatory. Keeping it in the bloodstream longer is extremely beneficial in the treatment of asthma, ulcers and intestinal inflammations and other chronic inflammatory conditions. In fact, licorice is used to gradually wean individuals off prednisone and other steroidal drugs in order to reestablish use of their own endogenous cortisone or to reduce dosages and protect the adrenal glands. Long-term treatment with steroids suppresses the natural production of endogenous corticosteroids from the adrenal glands and atrophies them. Sudden withdrawal of pharmaceutical steroids could lead to coma and death. (NOTE: *Never discontinue pharmaceutical steroids without the supervision of a physician.*) Herbal steroidal precursors do not stay in the body as long as pharmaceutical steroids. Therefore, even though an herb like licorice can lengthen cortisone's duration, its strength is still much less than a steroidal drug. This means that herbal steroids have neither the same strength nor the same serious side effects.

Yucca root contains saponins with reported cortisone-like activity which may explain its exceptional anti-inflammatory effects in arthritis. The saponins resemble steroidal hormones in chemistry and are used to produce the precursors of cortisone. Therefore, yucca may stimulate the adrenal glands to produce its own endogenous steroids. Yucca saponins resemble those of sarsaparilla, wild yam and fenugreek. Used by traditional peoples of both North and South America for relief of rheumatic pain, yucca root is a very useful anti-inflammatory for the treatment of both rheumatoid and osteoarthritis.[34] In fact, it has been used historically for inflammatory diseases of all kinds.

Sarsaparilla also contains steroidal saponins which exert anti-inflammatory effects. It may also work as an anti-inflammatory by enhancing endogenous steroid levels. It is particularly effective for conditions such as psoriasis, eczema, arthritis and ulcerative colitis since the steroid-like saponins bind to irritating gut endotoxins and remove them from circulation.

The Chinese herb *Rehmannia glutinosa* (the uncured form) appears to work as an anti-inflammatory by inhibiting the breakdown of cortisone and thereby extending its effects, like licorice. It also appears to counter adrenal atrophy caused by steroid hormones. In clinical studies it has been shown to alleviate the symptoms of asthma, hives and rheumatoid arthritis.[35]

Wild yam contains steroidal saponins such as diosgenin, which are believed to be responsible for its anti-inflammatory effects. It is especially effective for the whole gastrointestinal tract. It is used for irritable bowel syndrome (IBS), ulcerative colitis, ulcers, bowel inflammation, diverticulitis, cramping, intestinal colic and liver and gallbladder inflammation. Fenugreek also contains diosgenin and has been used historically as an anti-inflammatory agent.

It is also worth noting that vitamin C, which is used to form the adrenal corticosteroids, can help increase production of endogenous corticosteroids and improve the anti-inflammatory function of the body.

Triterpenoid Saponins. Bupleurum root is an important part of many traditional Chinese remedies. It has a long history of use for various conditions including allergies and other inflammatory conditions. It contains saikosaponins which have significant anti-inflammatory action and apparently increase the release of cortisone by the adrenal glands and help prevent adrenal gland atrophy due to steroid drug use. Licorice root and *Panax ginseng* are traditionally used with bupleurum root. They also contain triterpenoid saponins with anti-inflammatory activity that help protect the adrenal glands.

Gotu kola is very effective for reducing inflammation in connective tissue, veins and small blood vessels. It has been used in herbal medicine since prehistoric times in India and Indonesia to heal wounds. It has been reported to enhance connective tissue structure, stimulate regeneration of skin cells, reduce skin hardening (sclerosis) and to improve blood flow. Clinically it has been used to treat a variety of conditions, including wound healing, eczema, burns and scleroderma, with positive therapeutic results.

Guaiacum, a tree which grows in the Caribbean and South America, is primarily used for rheumatoid arthritis due to its potent anti-inflammatory action. In addition, it is used for osteoarthritis and other inflammatory processes.

The anti-inflammatory activity of black cohosh has been confirmed in a number of studies. In the early 19th century it had an excellent reputation as an anti-inflammatory for arthritis and rheumatism, and Native Americans also used the root for this purpose.

Calendula also contains saponins which have been linked with its anti-inflammatory action. It acts as a valuable digestive anti-inflammatory and is used in the treatment of gastric and duodenal ulcers, gastritis, colitis and diverticulitis.

ANTI-INFLAMMATORY VOLATILE OILS

Many aromatic volatile herbs have anti-inflammatory effects due to their essential oils. One of the best examples is chamomile, which contains a volatile oil that is high in the sequiterpenes alpha-bisabolol and chamazulene. Chamomile decreases histamine release and promotes wound healing. The essential oil, bisabolol, in chamomile has a strong anti-inflammatory action, is antibacterial and promotes skin granulation and tissue regeneration in wound repair. Bisabolol also decreases pepsin secretion in the stomach. In addition, chamomile is high in anti-inflammatory flavonoids and is particularly effective for eczema and gastrointestinal problems.

Calendula and St. John's wort are other herbs which contain essential oils that may play a part in their anti-inflammatory actions. St. John's wort oil is used externally for the treatment of wounds, abrasions and first-degree burns. Calendula is also used topically for treating inflammations, wounds, first-degree burns and sunburn.

Cinnamon, ginger and lavender also contain a volatile oil, cineole, which has been found to have antiallergy activity. In addition, celery seed contains a small percentage of volatile oils which appear to be effective for gout and arthritis. It also promotes the elimination of uric acid from the blood and assists the kidneys in clearing uric acid and other wastes from circulation. However, do not use celery seed during pregnancy or with kidney inflammation.

FLAVONOID-RICH PLANTS

Flavonoids, which are plant antioxidants, inhibit several in-flammatory chemical mediators including histamine, prostaglandins, leukotrines (by blocking lipoxygenase) and kinins. Flavonoids also decrease inflammation by desensitizing mast cells. For example, flavonoids such as baicalein from Chinese skullcap directly in-hibit the production of inflammatory mediators by stabilizing mast cells, and also inhibit enzymes in the arachidonic cascade such as lipoxygenases. Quercetin-rich herbs act to limit histamine release and other inflammatory chemicals. Other flavonoid-rich plants include pineapple (which also contains bromelain), calen-dula, turmeric, chamomile, St. John's wort ginkgo, bilberry, haw-thorn, elder berry, linden and milk thistle.

DEMULCENTS

True anti-inflammatories work on some level to inhibit the in-flammatory process by chemically mediating the products of inflammation. In contrast, demulcents soothe and protect tissues, but do not affect inflammatory metabolites at a cellular level. Therefore, many herbs listed as anti-inflammatories are merely demulcents. Marshmallow, for example, soothes and protects tissues. It is a demulcent; it does not directly inhibit the in-flammatory response. However these types of herbs are often referred to as anti-inflammatories in a general sense since they reduce local irritation.

OTHER TYPES OF HERBAL ANTI-INFLAMMATORIES

Other herbal anti-inflammatories work in multiple ways or through mechanisms not yet clearly understood. However, traditional therapeutic use has clearly established their effectiveness as anti-inflammatories. For example, herbalists around the world have used a number of other herbs to modify inflammation, such as bogbean, devil's claw and nettles. Herbalists know that these herbs work, but don't know exactly how. These traditional anti-inflammatory herbs will be discussed individually in the Concise Materia Medica.

Herbal Anti-Inflammatories for Different Body Sytems

Many anti-inflammatory herbs have a particular affinity to a specific body system. Utilizing herbs that are particularly suited to a specific body system tones, strengthens and revitalizes that area while also reducing any inflammation. The following are examples to consider, but this list is by no means conclusive.

Circulatory System. Herbs to reduce inflammation in the blood vessels include linden, hawthorn, horse chestnut, yarrow and bilberry.

Respiratory System. Herbs that reduce respiratory inflammation include licorice, gingko, feverfew, goldenrod, yerba santa, yerba mansa, eyebright, nettle, pleurisy root, coltsfoot, bupleurum root and oxeye daisy.

Digestive System. Herbs that reduce inflammation in the gastrointestinal system are particularly useful since herbs go directly to the digestive tract. These herbs include chamomile, wild yam, licorice, goldenseal, calendula and peppermint. In addition, sarsaparilla is effective for reducing inflammation in the gastrointestinal system since it binds endotoxins which are then more easily excreted from the body.

Urinary System. Herbs that soothe and reduce irritation in the urinary tract tissues include goldenrod and cornsilk. Uva ursi and cleavers are also effective urinary anti-inflammatories.

Reproductive System. Many reproductive tonics act as anti-inflammatories such as lady's mantle, blue cohosh and black cohosh.

Musculoskeletal System. The salicylate-containing herbs are particularly important, such as willow bark, meadowsweet and birch. In addition, other types of anti-inflammatories for these tissues that are specific for arthritis include bogbean, devil's claw, black cohosh, feverfew, wild yam, yucca root, chaparral, boswellia, *Commiphora mukul*, ashwagandha, guaiacum, nettle, turmeric, licorice, ginger, bromelain (from pineapple), celery seed, bupleurum root, sarsaparilla, yerba mansa and horsetail.

Integumentary (Skin) System. Herbs used externally that reduce inflammation on the skin include calendula, chamomile, St. John's wort, arnica, witch hazel, licorice and echinacea. Burdock, taken internally, also helps to reduce skin inflammation. Sarsaparilla reduces skin inflammations such as eczema and psoriasis by binding endotoxins. Gotu kola also has remarkable wound-healing activity and has been used to greatly aid wound repair and to relieve eczema.

Nervous System. Examples of anti-inflammatory herbs for the nervous system include St. John's wort, which also nourishes damaged nerves, Chinese skullcap as well as ashwagandha.

Let's take a closer look now at some common inflammatory conditions and apply these natural anti-inflammatory concepts.

Allergies and Asthma

Many people suffer from allergies and asthma. The underlying mechanisms and management are quite similar since they are both inflammatory in nature and have symptoms caused by the mediators of inflammation in the body. Asthma is primarily a condition of inflammation. It is essentially an allergic reaction that takes place in the bronchial airways of the lungs. Allergy is an inflammatory response to allergens, e.g., foods, chemicals, pollens or molds, and can result in asthma (wheezing and difficulty in breathing), sinus congestion with sneezing, itchy runny nose (hayfever), the itching and skin rash of hives and eczema, food-allergy diarrhea or migraine headaches. The unifying feature of all these allergy responses is the involvement of a specific group of antibodies (IgE) that attach to mast cells, primarily in the skin or the lining of the lungs, upper respiratory airways and stomach. These antibodies cause most cells to release histamine and other inflammatory chemicals when the allergen binds to them.

A natural approach to allergies or asthma involves:

◇ Decreasing exposure to the allergen.

◇ Toning down the overactive inflammatory response, preventing the formation and release of inflammatory mediators and preventing the breakdown of the body's own endogenous anti-inflammatory agents.

◇ Stimulating and supporting digestive processes to prevent the absorption of large dietary molecules leading to allergic responses.

◇ Soothing and improving mucous membrane integrity, normalizing mucus production and promoting expectoration to remove any excess mucus.

The goal is to rebalance the body so that susceptibility to the offending allergen is decreased. Herbal medicines should be part of a multi-faceted approach, however, and used along with other alternative strategies. Let's explore some of these specific strategies for addressing respiratory allergies and asthma.

CLEANING UP YOUR PERSONAL ENVIRONMENT

◇ Keep floors and carpets clean to reduce indoor pollutants. Vacuum cleaners should have an efficient filtering system so that allergens are not spread through the air. The use of ionizers or HEPA air purifiers can help remove pollen, dust and airborne allergenic substances. Alternatively, consider using more indoor houseplants as air purifiers.

◇ Do not allow pets to sleep in bedrooms if you have allergies or an allergic type of asthma.

◇ Keep bed sheets, mattress pads and pillowcases regularly cleaned. Consider using hypoallergenic synthetic bedding material.

◇ For chronic, ongoing allergies look for environmental causes and eliminate them. For example, dust, molds, cigarette smoke, feather pillows, smoke from wood stoves, etc. Smoking increases the risk of asthma by over 50 percent! If your child has asthma, do not allow others to smoke around them. Look for items that collect dust or molds such as rugs, draperies, upholstered furniture and eliminate them or keep them clean. Humidifier filters can also be a source of molds and bacteria, so either avoid their use or make sure filters are changed frequently.

◇ Use essential oil steams to help open congested nasal passages and enhance breakdown of mucus. Essential oils may also help open airways. Add approximately 5–8 drops of any of the following essential oils in a sink or pan of hot, steaming water: spruce, pine, eucalyptus, lavender, thyme, German chamomile, peppermint or rosemary. For asthma, a good combination is eucalyptus, peppermint and lavender. Make sure you use pure essential oils instead of synthetic fragrances. Form a towel tent over the pan or sink bowl and keep your head under the towel for 10 minutes. If the oils evaporate quickly, add an additional amount of 2–3 drops. Keep the face at least 18 inches away from the bowl to prevent burning and keep the eyes closed. Regulate the heat by raising or lowering the head or letting more air in from the outside.

As an alternative, place the essential oil of your choice on a washcloth and place it in the bottom of the shower before you turn the water on. While at work or traveling, keep a small bottle of essential oil in your pocket and inhale deeply a few times a day.

◇ Saline nasal washes are also effective in breaking down mucus associated with chronic runny noses and to clear nasal congestion. Place 1 tsp. of salt in 2 cups of warm water. The salt cuts the carbohydrate component of the nasal mucus and helps break down or thin out mucus. Take a bulk syringe filled with solution and squirt up into one side of the nose (or simply sniff solution up one nostril without using a bulb syringe), tilting the head to one side and inhaling the liquid up into the sinus. Hold for a few seconds and then exhale, allowing the liquid to drain into the sink. Then repeat for the other nostril. The herb, yerba mansa, can also be made into a tea, cooled off and added to the salt solution; it is often used in this way to treat allergic rhinitis or hay fever. Nasal congestion can cause postnasal drip which can increase the transport of inflammatory mediators from the nasal passages to the lungs and aggravate bronchial hyperreactivity. Thus, nasal washes and steams can be effective for both hay fever and asthma.

DIET

◇ Avoid dairy intake since dairy foods can thicken and increase mucus production. Avoid congestive foods such as processed foods and eat a wide variety of high-fiber foods, including whole grains, beans, vegetables and fruits. Avoid animal products, e.g., beef, poultry and dairy products, to reduce arachidonic acid and the inflammatory prostaglandins and leukotrienes it makes. Increase your consumption of cold-water fish, e.g., salmon, sardines and mackerel, and supplement with high-quality EPA supplements (2–3 g daily with meals) or flaxseed oil (1–2 Tbsp. daily) to help reduce inflammatory/allergic responses.

◇ Make sure to include onions and garlic in your diet since they both inhibit enzymes which generate inflammatory prostaglandins and leukotrienes.[36] Also, onion has shown an ability to prevent allergen-induced bronchial constriction.[37]

◇ Identify and avoid major food allergens. Persons with respiratory allergies may also have food allergies. Studies show that food allergies can play an important role in hay fever and asthma. Asthma can be triggered by almost any food allergen. Consider doing an elimination diet to identify your own allergens. For example, avoid dairy products for four weeks and see if you feel better. The most common allergenic foods include dairy, wheat, chocolate, peanuts, shellfish, corn, citrus fruits and juices, plus the food colorings and additives in foods. Tartrazine, EDTA derivatives, aspartame, MSG (monosodium glutamate), nitrates, formic acid, sorbic acid and benzoates are some of the major ones to look out for. It is also essential to avoid sulfites since they have been associated with triggering asthma attacks. Sulfite-containing foods include commercial baked goods, canned seafood, canned soups, frozen french fries, gelatin, beer, wine, vinegar, mushrooms, restaurant salads, maraschino cherries, dried fruits and sausage.

◇ Eat lots of whole natural foods, such as fruits and vegetables, preferably organically grown, since they are rich in antioxidants like vitamin C, carotenes and flavonoids which can protect against cellular damage and help quench the inflammatory response. Some people are allergic to citrus, so avoid if you are sensitive to it. Plus, drink green tea, which is another excellent antioxidant. It also reduces mast cell reactivity and secretion of histamine and other inflammatory chemicals and is believed to help open airways by acting as a bronchial dilator. Drink 1 cup every 3 hours, or a total of 5 cups daily, or take green tea extract supplements (200–300 mg 3 times daily).

◇ Optimize digestion to minimize absorbing large dietary molecules into the bloodstream and creating a reaction to foods. Use digestive enzymes, e.g., proteolytic enzymes, or use a little lemon juice with meals to stimulate pepsin production and to digest proteins more effectively.

◇ Drink lots of water to thin mucus secretions, to assist in detoxification and to act as a natural antihistamine. When the body becomes dehydrated, histamine production increases in an effort to hang on to existing water supplies. Drink at least 8–12 glasses of pure spring or distilled water daily. Drinking adequate amounts of water also protects against constipation, which can lead to toxins being reabsorbed from the bowel back into the bloodstream, aggravating allergies. If you are chronically constipated, try using a mild herbal laxative. A good Ayurvedic detoxification combination is trifala powder. Take 1 tsp. 1–2 times a day with a glass of water on a empty stomach.

◇ Adopt healthy dietary and lifestyle habits. Poor dietary habits, alcohol use, cigarette smoking and high levels of stress have been shown to increase allergic responses. For asthmatics, proper breathing exercises and stress reduction techniques are also helpful. Visualizations and relaxation techniques may be useful as well, particularly for children, to help manage fear during an attack.

◇ Reduce excessive dietary salt intake if you are asthmatic, since it has been found that the greater the intake of salt, the more reactive the bronchial tubes are to histamine.[38]

NUTRITIONAL SUPPLEMENTS

Quercetin is a bioflavonoid found extensively in foods and in many herbs, including hawthorn, chamomile, calendula, gingko, elder and linden flowers. It is also available in a concentrated supplement form. It is a potent anti-inflammatory and has been shown to be a potent inhibitor of mast cell and basophil degranulation.[39] Since the release of histamine and other inflammatory compounds from mast cells and basophils are involved in inflammatory allergic responses, quercetin is specifically indicated for allergies and asthma. Like other bioflavonoids, it is a natural antihistamine. In addition, it is a potent antioxidant which neutralizes free radicals and prevents the formation of inflammatory mediators like leukotrienes. However, quercetin may not be well absorbed by the body; combining it with bromelain (the anti-inflammatory enzyme from pineapple) may enhance its absorption. The suggested supplement dosage for an adult is 250–500 mg of each, 20 minutes before meals on an empty stomach or in-between meals, 2–3 times daily.

Other Antioxidants are also important for relieving asthma since free radicals not only stimulate airway constriction but increase allergic reactions to other agents.[40] Potent antioxidant supplements such as proanthocyanidins (extracted from grape seed and pine bark) and curcumin from turmeric should also be considered to neutralize free radicals and help quench the inflammatory response. Proanthocyanidins have been shown to prevent the release and formation of mediators that cause inflammation, including histamine, prostaglandins and leukotrienes.[41] The recommended dosage for grape seed or pine bark extract is 50–100 mg 3 times per day.

Vitamin C, E and Selenium. Vitamin C is another important antioxidant which can decrease histamine levels and provide anti-inflammatory action.[42] The recommended dosage is 3,000–5,000 mg daily. Vitamin C can cause diarrhea in some people, so either cut the dosage back to a level where symptoms disappear or use buffered C if you have stomach problems or discomfort. In addition, the antioxidants vitamin E (400 IU daily) and selenium (50–200 mcg daily) have also demonstrated antiallergy effects.[43]

Beta-carotene is a carotenoid which helps regenerate the epithelial lining of the nose and throat, healing and soothing irritated mucous membranes. As an antioxidant, it also helps quench the inflammatory process by neutralizing free radicals. The recommended dosage for beta-carotene is 25,000–50,000 IU daily. Unlike vitamin A, which should not be taken in doses greater than 25,000 IU for extended periods of time due to its potential for cumulative toxicity, beta-carotene, which is the precursor of vitamin A, can be taken in higher doses for prolonged periods of time without toxicity.

Magnesium supplementation is recommended to reduce bronchial constriction and improve asthmatic breathing. The dose is 500–750 mg daily of magnesium chelate or aspartate. It relaxes muscles and rapidly opens bronchial tubes without side effects.[44]

B Vitamins. Vitamin B6 (pyridoxine) also decreases the frequency and severity of symptoms related to air bound allergies and vitamin B12 is a mainstay in asthma and also useful in hayfever.[45]

HERBAL TREATMENTS

Treatment for allergies and asthma has a lot to do with the inflammatory effects of the substances being released by mast cells. When an allergen binds to an antibody (IgE) that is attached to a mast cell, it causes the cell to release its inflammatory contents, such as histamine, chemotactic factors, leukotrienes, and prostaglandins. Leukotrienes contribute to bronchial spasms in asthma by narrowing the airways and causing excess mucus production; prostaglandins contribute to constriction and bronchial spasm; histamines cause swelling (due to increased permeability of blood vessels and more liquid moving into the space), stimulate secretion of large amounts of mucus and constrict the respiratory passages, causing the familiar symptoms of allergies such as runny nose; itchy, watery eyes; sneezing and a stuffy, congested nose.

Thus, in asthma, in addition to anti-inflammatory remedies, antispasmodic and expectorant herbs are also helpful for bronchial dilation and mucus resolution. However, it should be noted that these approaches are not generally recommended for acute asthma attacks. Herbal treatments for acute attacks should be undertaken under the guidance of a skilled practitioner. Those who are using metered-dose inhalers for asthma can still use herbal remedies; however, working with a naturopathic physician or medical herbalist who is trained in the multifaceted approaches to asthma is the optimal solution.

In hay fever, in addition to anti-inflammatory herbs, decongestant, anticatarrhal and astringent herbs are also used. Herbs, due to their gentle but effective actions, can alleviate symptoms without causing rebound symptoms. If used correctly, there is neither toxicity or negative side effects. This is in stark contrast to most mainstream drugs for asthma and allergies.

The following are primary herbs to try. For more detailed information and dosages, consult the Concise Materia Medica beginning on page 93.

Licorice slows the breakdown of our own natural cortisone and is one of the key herbs for allergy and asthma treatment due to its cortisone enhancing anti-inflammatory actions. It helps block the release of histamine and serotonin from mast cells and helps maintain the integrity of the mast cell membrane, stabilizing it and making it less likely to spill out chemicals. Licorice also inhibits the enzyme responsible for releasing arachidonic acid from its storage site in cell membranes, leading to the formation of inflammatory prostaglandins. In addition, licorice enhances the production of suppressor T-cells, reducing the immune response to allergens.

Ginkgo is very useful for people with allergies and asthma because it inhibits the actions of PAF, a major chemical mediator in asthma, inflammation and allergies. In addition, gingko contains flavones and quercetin and is a good antioxidant, which add to its anti-inflammatory effects. Other botanicals which inhibit PAF include ginger and turmeric, among others.

Hawthorn blocks the enzyme that converts histadine to histamine, so it is particularly useful in allergies and histamine-type reactions. It is also high in flavonoids, including quercetin.

Feverfew is another effective anti-inflammatory to consider for allergies and asthma. Feverfew inhibits the enzyme responsible for releasing arachidonic acid, which forms inflammatory prostaglandins and leukotrienes. It also inhibits degranulation and re-

69

lease of histamine, serotonin and other inflammatory mediators from mast cells.

Ephedra or ma-huang has a long traditional use in the treatment of allergies, hay fever and asthma, specifically relieving the bronchoconstriction associated with asthma. It has been used to treat asthma in China for over 2,000 years. The herb is also excellent as a decongestant in hay fever and reduces allergic reactions.

Tylophora is an Ayurvedic herb used extensively in asthma and other respiratory tract disorders. It has been reported to possess antihistamine activity, antispasmodic activity and to inhibit mast cell degranulation, thereby preventing the release of inflammatory mediators.

Chinese skullcap is an excellent anti-inflammatory herb. It inhibits the release of histamine from mast cells and as such is very useful in the treatment of allergies and asthma that has an allergic component to it. In addition, it appears to gently inhibit the bronchoconstriction associated with asthma.

Nettle has been successfully used in the treatment of hay fever and allergies.

Goldenrod is specific for relieving upper respiratory congestion. Its actions are anticatarrhal, anti-inflammatory, antimicrobial, astringent and diuretic. It thins secretions, making them easier to get rid of, and it slows down the production of mucus.

Lobelia is often used to treat spasmodic asthma and is extremely beneficial; however, it can cause nausea and vomiting in high doses. Lobelia, along with licorice and ginkgo, is helpful to keep the lungs free from excessive mucus.

Skunk cabbage is indicated for asthma sufferers who expectorate alot. It is an expectorant and respiratory sedative that has strong antispasmodic effects on the respiratory passages.

Dong quai inhibits platelet aggregation and has anti-inflammatory action. It has been used by Chinese herbalists to prevent and relieve allergy symptoms.

Reishi mushroom also has antiallergy effects due to its ability to inhibit histamine release and leukotriene production. Start taking as soon as the hayfever season begins—1000 mg, three times daily.

Bupleurum root has significant anti-inflammatory action and is specifically indicated for allergies.

Boswellia is another excellent anti-inflammatory for bronchial asthma and ashwaghanda, another ayurvedic herb, is also commonly used for asthma, especially for children.

Other Western Herbs Used for Asthma

Elecampane is a stimulating expectorant specific for chronic mucus and wet cough. It is also a carminative, diuretic and astringent.

Grindelia, a commonly used herb for bronchial asthma, is a stimulating expectorant and antispasmodic.

Mullein is indicated for asthma, hay fever, bronchitis and dry coughs. It is a soothing demulcent, sedative expectorant and anti-inflammatory that helps rid the lungs of congestion.

Other Western Herbs Used for Allergies:

Eyebright which has anti-inflammatory, anticatarrhal and astringent properties.

Sage is anticatarrhal, mildly expectorating and a good decongestant.

Yerba mansa is particularly good for subacute congestions in the mucous membranes and useful for congestion in the respiratory membranes.

Yerba santa is a resinous stimulating expectorant, bronchiodilator and decongestant.

Elder flower is an anticatarrhal expectorant and astringent to the mucous membranes of the nose, sinuses and bronchioles.

Goldenseal is an anticatarrhal, anti-inflammatory, antimicrobial, astringent and expectorant specific to the mucous membranes which is also high in flavonoids.

Canadian fleabane is useful in all types of congestion, including hay fever.

General Herbal Formulas for Asthma and Allergies

I. Lobelia Compound

This asthma formula, created by Tieraona Low Dog, M.D., and designed to enhance bronchodilation, reduce inflammation and assist expectoration, is available through Materia Medica herb company (see Resources). It is a blend of ephedra, licorice root, Chinese skullcap, dry lobelia and capsicum.

II. Asthma Formula

Mix the following tinctures: 6 tsp. each of ephedra herb and ginkgo leaf; 3 tsp. each of cramp bark, mullein leaf and dried lobelia herb.

Dosage: 60–80 drops of the blend in hot water, 2–3 times per day for adults; 30–60 drops in hot water 2–3 times per day for children. It is best taken with standardized extract of gingko (80 mg 3 times per day), vitamin C (3,000–5,000 mg per day) and licorice root 1:1 extract (½ tsp. 3 times per day not to exceed 6 weeks).

III. Allergy Formula

Blend the following tinctures: 6 tsp. each of ginkgo leaf and whole ephedra herb plus 5 tsp. each of yerba santa leaf and goldenrod herb.

Take 1 tsp. of the blend in hot water, 3 times daily. For chronic, ongoing symptoms take ½ tsp. in hot water 3–4 times daily.

IV. David Hoffmann's Allergy Formula[46]

Blend the following tinctures together and take 1 tsp., 3 times a day: 1 part each Chinese ephedra, goldenseal and eyebright; 2 parts each nettle and goldenrod. If this is used for seasonal allergies, start it two months before the season begins and take throughout the season.

V. Herbal Tea for Hay Fever

Combine and mix well: 2 parts elder flowers plus 1 part each ephedra stems, eyebright herb/aerial parts, nettle herb and goldenseal root.

To make 1 quart of tea, pour 4 cups of boiling water over 2 Tbsp. of the herb mixture, cover and allow to sit for 10–15 minutes. Strain and serve. Drink 1 cup 3 times a day.

Note: For all formulas listed above containing ephedra or lobelia, read the contraindications listed in the Concise Materia Medica.

Rheumatoid Arthritis

Arthritis means joint inflammation. Rheumatoid arthritis is a common form of joint inflammation that is chronic. The disease targets the inner linings of the joint capsules, especially those in the hands, feet, wrists, ankles and knees, causing them to become inflamed. The inflammation is the result of an immune reaction against the body's own tissues such that the body attacks and damages joints, surrounding connective tissue and cartilage. Although the exact causes of this autoimmune process are not known, the possibilities include genetic predisposition, viral infection, abnormal bowel permeability (leaky gut syndrome), susceptibility to food allergies, lifestyle and dietary factors. Food allergies are believed to play a significant role in the inflammatory process. They damage intestinal membranes, resulting in abnormal bowel permeability allowing toxins and immune complexes to leak into the body.

Traditional treatment usually includes nonsteroidal anti-inflammatory drugs (NSAIDs), corticosteroids, surgical repair or replacement of damaged joints. Unfortunately, these treatments can have many adverse side effects. NSAIDs can even inhibit cartilage repair and accelerate cartilage destruction and progression of the disease. Although rheumatoid arthritis is a complex disease, natural medicine, including the use of herbs, can help to extend periods of remission and ease inflammation and pain without adverse side effects.

DIETARY FACTORS

Eliminate allergenic foods. Common offenders include wheat, corn, dairy products, red meat and foods in the nightshade family (tomatoes, eggplant, potatoes, peppers). Juice fasts or therapeutic fasting followed by a vegetarian diet have been effective in reducing disease activity; however, be sure to consult with a qualified health practitioner before starting any type of fasting. It is believed that vegetarian diets are effective since they decrease the amount of arachidonic acid in the diet, which is responsible for the production of inflammatory prostaglandins. Eating cold-water fish such as mackerel, herring, sardines and salmon or supplementing the diet with 2–3g of omega-3 EPA oils daily with meals have also shown a significant reduction in inflammation. Eating flavonoid-rich foods, such as cherries, blueberries and other dark red-blue berries rich in anthocyanidins and proanthocyanidins also can help prevent destruction of joint tissues.

NUTRIENTS

Antioxidants are very important since much of the joint destruction is due to free radical damage. These include vitamin C

(3,000 mg daily or as tolerated), selenium (50–200 mcg daily) and vitamin E (400 IU daily). The nutrients zinc (30 mg daily) and manganese (5–15 mg daily) are also important in helping increase antioxidant activity. In addition, flavonoids such as quercetin (250–600 mg daily) are important in inhibiting the production and release of inflammatory chemicals as well as curcumin, another powerful antioxidant which may be one of nature's most potent anti-inflammatories. Take curcumin combined with bromelain (400–600 mg of each, 3 times daily, between meals). Proteolytic enzymes such as bromelain are important in reducing swelling and helping to eliminate immune complexes that have been deposited in the joints. Digestive enzymes, e.g., 10x USP pancreatic enzyme preparations, and hydrochloric acid (HCL) taken with meals also help improve digestion and reduce food allergy sensitivities. However, before beginning HCL supplementation, first have your health practitioner test to determine need. Alternatively, take bitter digestive herbs to stimulate digestion (e.g. dandelion root, yellow dock root, barberry root bark and chamomile).

Herbal Treatments

The following anti-inflammatory herbs have shown positive effects in the management of rheumatoid arthritis: licorice, bupleurum root, turmeric (curcumin), Chinese skullcap, *Rehmannia glutinosa*, willow bark, meadowsweet, bogbean, devil's claw, black cohosh, feverfew, yucca root, chaparral, yerba mansa, boswellia, *Commiphora mukul*, ashwagandha, guaiacum, nettle, ginger,

celery seed, wild yam and sarsaparilla. For more detailed information and dosages, consult the Concise Materia Medica beginning on page 93. In addition, flavonoid-rich herbs such as
hawthorn and bilberry have collagen-healing properties indicated for damaged cartilage as well as antioxidant actions. Herbs
like horsetail and gotu kola stimulate tissue repair and would
also be useful in increasing the repair and regeneration of connective tissue. These herbs, used individually or preferably in
combination, are indicated for rheumatoid arthritis. In preparing
a formula, consider herbs with the following herbal actions that
are specific for arthritis:

Anti-inflammatory herbs to address the inflammatory nature of
the disease (e.g. licorice, feverfew, devil's claw, bupleurum root,
Chinese skullcap, wild yam, guaiacum, *Rhemannia glutinosa*, black
cohosh, yucca root, boswellia, turmeric, *Commiphora mukul*, ginger, ashwagandha, chaparral and willow).

Alteratives to help restore proper metabolism and to strengthen
overall vitality (e.g. nettles, guaiacum, bogbean, burdock,
prickly ash, alfalfa and sarsaparilla).

Circulatory stimulants (e.g. prickly ash, ginger, guaiacum), **diuretics** (e.g. celery seed, yerba mansa, nettles), **mild laxatives**
(e.g. dandelion root) to enhance elimination.

Bitter liver herbs to stimulate digestion and detoxify the liver
(e.g. bogbean, dandelion root, barberry).

78

Many herbalists believe that results are better when each herb in a formula is within its own therapeutic dose range; therefore, using fewer herbs in therapeutic dosages rather than many herbs in subtherapeutic doses may be more effective.

Herbal Arthritis Formulas

I. Blend the following tinctures: 5 tsp. each of guaiacum, devil's claw and celery seed; 4 tsp. of willow bark and licorice; 2 tsp. of feverfew.
Dosage: Take 1–2 tsp. (in water or juice if desired) before each meal.

II. Mix the following tinctures in equal parts: *Rhemannia glutinosa,* bupleurum root, feverfew and licorice.
Dosage: Take 1–2 tsp. (in water or juice if desired) 3 times daily.
Note: See contraindications and cautions for licorice root in the Concise Materia Medica, p. 113–115.

III. **Tea Formula:** 2 parts nettles, dandelion root and willow bark; 1 part ginger root; ½ part prickly ash bark. Mix thoroughly and place 1 tsp. in a cup of boiling water for 15–20 minutes. Drink 3 cups per day.

The guidance of a qualified herbalist or naturopathic physician in selecting an individualized formula is recommended for optimum results.

ADDITIONAL SUGGESTIONS

Physical therapy can play a significant role in improving joint mobility and reducing pain. Modalities include appropriate exercise, hot and cold compresses, showers or baths to stimulate general circulation, massage, paraffin baths and shortwave diathermy. Topical analgesic salves containing cayenne pepper can be used to block the transmission of pain impulses but only as a supportive measure combined with other deeper-acting approaches. Lastly, stress appears to affect the disease process, so stress reduction and relaxation exercises may also be beneficial along with herbs to soothe the nerves and reduce stress. For example, St. John's wort, chamomile, kava kava, linden, passionflower or lemon balm would be excellent nervines to consider for stress. Acupuncture can also be very beneficial in arthritis for reduction of pain and plays an important role in holistic treatment since it helps re-establish stressed or imbalanced organ systems by stimulating the flow of energy through meridians.

The severity of rheumatoid arthritis varies from person to person and can range from mild to severe. Mild to moderate cases respond well to the natural approaches listed above and even severe cases requiring drug therapy can benefit, making it possible to reduce required drug doses. Chronic diseases often require long-term compliance and vigilance. Changes can be gradual and take months, but positive results are possible with dietary, lifestyle, nutritional and herbal approaches.

Inflammatory Bowel Diseases

Crohn's disease and ulcerative colitis are the two major forms of chronic inflammatory disease (IBD). Crohn's disease usually affects the ileum or last portion of the small intestine but can also affect any part of the GI tract from mouth to rectum. Ulcerative colitis is limited to the colon. The exact cause is not known but several different theories include genetic predisposition, microbial agents, dietary factors, including food allergies, immune system dysfunction and psychological factors. However, diet may be one of the most important factors.

DIET AND NUTRITION

Inflammation is central to both of these disorders, which are characterized by diarrhea (sometimes bloody), malabsorption of nutrients and intestinal pain. These conditions can be described as allergic reactions in the intestines with greatly increased prostaglandin levels present in the affected tissues. Thus, dietary

81

sources of arachidonic acid should be reduced and omega-3 oils such as flaxseed oil and fish oils (EPA) should be added to the diet as in other inflammatory conditions. In addition, one of the first considerations is to avoid allergenic foods since food sensitivities appear to exacerbate the disease. Some common allergenic foods include wheat, corn and dairy products.

Other measures include a high-fiber, low refined-carbohydrate and low-sugar diet; however, initially the colon may be so irritated that fiber might aggravate the symptoms. Thus, high-fiber foods must be introduced slowly. Water-soluble fiber, e.g., psyllium, pectin, guar gum, etc., taken at bedtime, can assist in adding bulk, regulating bowel function and binding irritating bowel toxins. In addition, probiotics, such as lactobacillus acidophilus and bifidobacteria supplementation will help reestablish the healthy intestinal flora often outnumbered by high levels of toxic intestinal bacteria in patients with IBD.

Nutritional complications are common, and correcting these is very important in management of the disease. Nutritional deficiencies, inadequate calorie intake and low protein levels all need to be addressed. Nutritional supplements recommended include magnesium chelates, e.g., citrate or aspartate, 200 mg 3 times daily, vitamin E (400 IU daily), Vitamin D (100-400 IU daily), mycelized vitamin A (25,000 IU daily—high doses can be toxic so do not exceed), zinc picolinate (50 mg daily), quercetin (250–500 mg with an equal amount of bromelain), vitamin B12 (1,000 mcg daily), folic acid (1 mg daily), vitamin C (3,000 mg daily or as tolerated; use with caution in acute phases where it may irritate intestinal mucosa), selenium (50–200 mcg daily) and digestive enzymes as discussed previously. Quercetin is particularly indicated since it not only has antioxidant activity but also inhibits the release of histamine and other inflammatory chemicals, thereby reducing food allergies and the inflammatory response in the bowel. Other antioxidants such as grape seed extract, green tea and curcumin are also recommended. Take as directed on product labels. People with IBD are also prone to developing vitamin K deficiencies. Vitamin K is vital for proper blood clotting and is found in blue green algae supplements and fat soluable chlorophyll preparations. Take as directed. Freeze dried nettle capsules or fresh nettle leaf tea is also an excellent source of vitamin K along with all dark green leafy vegetables.

It cannot be overemphasized that IBD is a complex disease which can have serious consequences and requires the care and guidance of a qualified health care professional. An individualized diet and nutritional program by a trained professional is very important for everyone with IBD.

HERBAL TREATMENTS

Many herbs used historically for IBD are demulcents or mucilaginous herbs such as marshmallow root, slippery elm bark or plantain. Demulcents soothe irritated or inflamed internal tissues and promote mucus secretion, an effect indicated by a decrease in intestinal mucus production in proportion to disease severity.

Chamomile and calendula have also been used traditionally for inflammatory bowel disorders. They can be taken frequently throughout the day as teas to protect and heal intestinal mucosa.

These herbs are anti-inflammatories and antioxidants high in flavonoids, which are specifically indicated since they decrease the release of inflammatory mediators.

A significant correlation exists between free radical activity in the intestines and IBD activity;[47] thus, antioxidants play an important role. Sulfasalazine, the most widely prescribed drug for IBD, has been shown to inhibit the activity of free radicals;[48] unfortunately, it also inhibits the absorption and metabolism of folate, decreases folate and iron levels and increases urinary excretion of vitamin C. Other adverse side effects include hypersensitivity reactions. Herbal and nutritional antioxidants on the other hand, have no adverse side effects. Herbs high in flavonoids which are antioxidants include calendula, chamomile, tumeric, bilberry and hawthorn. Flavonid rich herbs are also indicated since capillary bleeding is usually involved and flavonoids increase the integrity of the blood vessel walls and reduce capillary fragility.

Antimicrobials such as oregon grape and goldenseal (specific to mucous membranes) are effective in inhibiting toxic bacterial growth. Echinacea is also useful since it has both anti-inflammatory and antimicrobial activity. Wild yam, which is an anti-inflammatory and antispasmodic, can help alleviate inflammation and cramps. Fenugreek is another herbal remedy to consider since it possesses anti-inflammatory, demulcent and antispasmodic actions. Mild astringents, such as raspberry, yarrow, Canadian fleabane, agrimony or cranesbill, help prevent bleeding and protect from further irritation. Licorice root is a useful anti-inflammatory herb to consider also since it possesses demulcent and antispasmodic properties. Another anti-inflammatory herb, sarsaparilla, is specifically indicated since it binds intestinal endotoxins which can be more easily excreted from the body.

Again, stress appears to adversely affect the disease process so practice stress reduction and use herbal nervines such as chamomile, kava kava, St. John's wort, lemon balm, passion flower and linden. Linden is an excellent remedy for stress, is antispasmodic, mildly astringent for diarrhea and high in flavonoids (especially quercetin). Lemon balm is also antispasmodic, high in flavonoids and useful for over anxiety that causes digestive tract problems. Lemon balm lifts the spirits and is referred to traditionally as the "gladdening herb". These herbal nervines calm the central nervous system without the addictive or overly sedating effects found in tranquilizing drugs. In addition, as with all chronic disease processes, herbal adaptogens are indicated to help deal with prolonged stress. For example, reishi, ashwagandha, astragalus and siberian ginseng are all very helpful in increasing the body's resistance to stress.

Also, higher than normal levels of leukotrienes are found in the mucosa of those suffering from inflammatory bowel disease so herbs that inhibit the leukotriene pathway, in which lipoxygenase is the key enzyme, are particularly useful and include boswellia, Chinese skullcap and other flavonoid rich herbs.

IBS Herbal Tea Blend

Mix the following herbs in equal proportions: licorice root, slippery elm, marshmallow root, red raspberry leaf and chamomile. To make 1 quart of tea, place 3 Tbsp. of chopped, mixed herbs into 4 cups of boiling water and simmer gently for 10–15 minutes. Fenugreek seeds can also be added to the tea. Add an additional cup of water and before simmering adds 5 tsp. of seeds. However, they are somewhat bitter so also adding 1-2 tsp. of anise seeds makes the tea more palatable. Strain and serve warm (not hot). Drink 1 cup 3 times a day. See contraindications in the Concise Materia Medica for licorice.

Robert's Formula for IBD

Robert's formula is an old herbal remedy that has been used in treating IBD. The formula includes marshmallow (demulcent); wild indigo (antimicrobial for GI infections); echinacea (antimicrobial, immune stimulant, anti-inflammatory); cranesbill (astringent to control bleeding); goldenseal (antimicrobial and mucous membrane tonic); poke root (promotes healing of intestinal ulcerations—toxic in large doses); comfrey (anti-inflammatory and wound healer, generally not for internal use due to potential liver toxicity with prolonged use); slippery elm (demulcent). A modified version of this formula which does not contain poke root, comfrey or wild indigo, manufactured by Enzymatic Therapy, is available in health food stores.

Eczema

Eczema is a chronic inflammatory skin condition usually called dermatitis. Many different types of eczema exist depending on their causes, location and appearance. There are various causes, but generally eczema can be defined as a severe allergic reaction manifesting on the skin; it often accompanies hay fever and asthma. Eczema is usually the end result of a series of internal reactions due to allergen exposure. There is evidence of abnormal bowel permeability as found in leaky gut syndrome. Thus similar factors are present in eczema as in rheumatoid arthritis and asthma—such as food allergies, fewer stomach secretions, which are needed for proper digestion, and an imbalance in fatty acids resulting in inflammatory compounds.

The naturopathic view is that eczema is the result of a disruption in normal functioning of the digestive system, liver, immune system, nervous system and skin. Factors that can cause this disruption include food allergies, environmental sensitivities, emotional stress, irritants and genetic predisposition. The treatment goals are to eliminate food allergens; inhibit the allergic response by reducing inflammation; reduce environmental sensitivity; reduce emotional stress; improve digestive, liver, lym-

87

phatic and immune system functioning, and support skin healing. The skin is one of the ways the body eliminates waste products. When the detoxifying and eliminative systems function properly, the skin can perform its eliminative function without causing skin irritation or eruptions. However, when toxins accumulate and other systems are overloaded or deficient, then the skin's elimination role manifests as skin eruptions, scaling and rashes, as with eczema. Thus, eczema is best treated internally.

DIET AND NUTRITION

Diet can play an important role in the management of eczema since it is, at least partially, caused by allergy. Thus, eliminating food allergens is one of the first steps. The best way to determine food allergens is by an elimination diet. Eliminate the suspected allergen for four weeks and then reintroduce and assess the result. Common food allergens include wheat (gluten-containing), dairy (milk and all milk products), shellfish and citrus fruits. Gluten allergies are common and include foods such as barley, rye, oats and wheat (think BROW). Allergies to food additives are also common, so avoid as much as possible. Eat a varied diet, rotating foods to assess benefit. Eat whole foods, including vegetables, especially those rich in beta-carotene, such as carrots, winter squash and leafy greens. Also, consume cold-water fish high in omega-3 fatty acids such as salmon, mackerel or sardines. Avoid arachidonic acid found in animal foods since it gives rise to inflammatory products. Eczema may be the result of an omega-3 fatty acid deficiency so supplementation with EPA-rich fish oils is highly recommended. Plus, drink several cups of green tea throughout the day to inhibit allergic mechanisms.

Many people with eczema also have low levels of hydrochloric acid (HCL) in their stomachs. The lower the level, the worse the eczema is. Thus, supplementation with HCL as well as other digestive enzymes may be beneficial to properly break down food.

Nutrients recommended for eczema include fish oil supplements (2–3g of EPA daily with meals) or evening primrose oil (4–6g daily), zinc picolinate (30–50 mg 3 times a day), vitamin E (400 IU daily), mycelized vitamin A (25,000 IU daily), vitamin C (3.5–5g daily or as tolerated), bioflavonoids (500 mg daily), and quercetin/bromelain combination (250–500 mg of each, 15–30 minutes before meals)

HERBAL TREATMENTS

Many herbs have demonstrated excellent results in the treatment of eczema. Herbal actions indicated for the processes behind this disease include:

Alteratives to assist detoxification: red clover, nettles, cleavers, burdock, sarsaparilla, calendula.

Anti-inflammatories to inhibit allergic responses and reduce inflammation: licorice, sarsaparilla, chamomile, ginkgo, Chinese skullcap, feverfew, turmeric.

Lymphatic tonics to improve waste elimination through the lymphatic system: cleavers.

Diuretics to ensure adequate elimination through the kidneys: cleavers, yarrow.

Bitter digestive stimulants and **liver detoxicants** to improve digestive functioning and improve liver function: milk thistle, dandelion root, yellow dock, oregon grape, burdock.

Nervines to address the associated problems of anxiety and stress: skullcap, chamomile, lemon balm, St. John's wort, linden, passion flower and kava kava.

Antimicrobials to help control bacterial staph infections in the skin, which are common in eczema: echinacea, goldenseal, burdock.

Other herbs to consider when preparing a formula in addition to the above are flavonoid-rich herbs that reduce histamine production and secretion, such as bilberry, hawthorn and ginkgo. Gotu kola is another useful herb for eczema. It enhances tissue regeneration, especailly connective tissue. Other herbs which are specifically indicated for eczema include boswellia, *Commiphora mukul*, turmeric, Chinese skullcap and other flavonoid rich herbs which reduce elevated leukotriene levels associated with eczema.

In addition, a number of herbal topical applications can be used in place of cortisone which when used long term makes the skin fragile and weak, increasing susceptibility to infection and damage. Licorice, when applied to the skin, has similar effects to cortisone but without negative side effects. Licorice compresses applied cool help relieve inflammation and itching. Dip a compress cloth in cool licorice tea and apply to the affected area. Avoid hot compresses on hot inflamed tissue. Also avoid long hot baths, which dehydrate the skin, and apply adequate moisturizers specifically for hypersensitive skin; zinc oxide applied locally helps relieve the severe itchiness of eczema. Oatmeal baths made by using bath powders like Aveeno also help relieve itching. Chamomile is also very effective topically providing symptomatic relief to the skin. Other herbs for topical use include chickweed (itching relief), calendula (anti-inflammatory and wound healing), witch hazel (anti-inflammatory and relieves itching), comfrey (wound healing) and St. John's wort (anti-inflammatory). Simicort cream by Enzymatic Therapy is an effective combination which includes chamomile, licorice and allantoin. However, skin problems can be successfully addressed only from within, using internal remedies; topical applications are merely supportive.

Herbal Eczema Formulas

Tincture I: Blend equal parts of burdock, cleavers, sarsaparilla, oregon grape and yellow dock. Take 1–2 tsp. 3 times a day. Reduced dosages may be necessary to avoid an initial symptomatic crisis caused by releasing large amounts of toxic substances from the tissues into the bloodstream. Burdock is a powerful detoxifying herb and, unless the eliminatory organs are functioning properly, an initial crisis may result.

Tincture II: Blend equal parts of oregon grape, licorice and echinacea. Take 2 tsp. 3–4 times per day for 6 weeks; then remove the licorice and substitute with another anti-inflammatory herb, such as ginkgo which blocks PAF, a key inflammatory mediator in eczema. See contraindications in the Concise Materia Medica for licorice. Echinacea may be used alone, especially for children who scratch and develop secondary infections. Take 1 tsp. 3–4 times a day for 6 weeks.

Tea: Blend equal parts of red clover, cleavers, nettle and chamomile. Pour 1 cup boiling water over 2-3 tsp.'s of mixed herbs and steep for 15 minutes. Strain and drink 3–4 cups per day. Another wonderful tea for eczema, especially for children, is burdock, nettle. For every 1 cup of water add 1 tsp. burdock root and bring to a boil, simmering gently for 10 minutes; remove from heat and add 1 tsp. nettle leaves for each cup of water used then cover and allow to sit for 10 minutes; strain and drink 2-3 cups per day.

Traditionally, formulas are taken regularly over an extended period of time. As with other inflammatory conditions when treating eczema with herbs, clinical effects may take several months. The results are rewarding, however, and go to the root of the problem, giving increased vitality and health to the whole body.

Concise Materia Medica

Primary herbal anti-inflammatories and selected supportive herbs used in inflammatory conditions mentioned throughout this book are concisely described here. For other herbs not in this Materia Medica check the Appendix, pp. 129-131, for latin names and part used.

The dosages listed are per day, for a 150 pound person and represent an average effective dose. For those with weights significantly more or less than this, there are several rules that can be used to adjust the dose. For example, Clark's rule takes the weight of the person, divides it by 150 to give the fraction of the adult dose to be used. Thus, a woman weighing 120 pounds would take 120/150 or ⅘ths of the adult dose.

ARNICA   *Arnica montana, A. latifolia, and A. cordifolia*

Part used: Flowers, sometimes roots.

Actions: Anti-inflammatory, vulnerary, stimulant.

Therapeutics: Superior remedy for external local healing, specifically for bruises, sprains, strains, muscle pain and soreness. Arnica improves local blood supply, speeds healing and increases the rate of reabsorption of internal bleeding, enhancing resolution. Do not use arnica on broken skin and *do not take this herb internallly,* only the homeoptahic preparation is appropriate for internal use.

Dosage: Apply diluted tincture directly to affected area or make a compress of arnica tea or diluted tincture on a cloth; apply freely to loosen tight muscles or to soothe inflammation. Reapply every 1–2 hours or as needed. Discontinue use if skin irritation or rash develops. Arnica may also be applied as a salve or cream.

Contraindications: Arnica allergy. In prolonged treatment of damaged skin, e.g., in injuries or leg ulcers, potential dermatitis with blistering can occur.

BILBERRY   *Vaccinium myrtillus*

Part used: Ripe fruit (berries), leaves.

Actions: Anti-inflammatory, vascular stabilizer, microcirculation enhancer, antioxidant.

Therapeutics: Flavonoids are bilberry's active constituents, specifically anthocyanosides, which are powerful antioxidants that protect and strengthen capillaries by preventing free radical damage. In addition, they stimulate formation of collagen in healthy connective tissue formation and aid in new capillary formation. Bilberry may also reduce platelet aggregation. It has been used widely in the treatment of vascular disorders and in eye conditions such as night blindness and diabetic retinopathy.

It promotes healthy circulation throughout the body and may also be considered to assist healing following surgery or traumatic injury. Weak capillaries or capillary fragility can lead to poor blood circulation to connective tissues throughout the body, hindering healing of tissue as occurs in trauma or inflammatory conditions such as arthritis. Bilberry enhances the formation of healthy connective tissue by promoting cross-linking of collagen, thus it is particularly useful in protecting connective tissue from damage secondary to inflammation and assists in the regeneration of normal connective tissue after injury.

Dosage: Standardized products: 240–480 mg daily, divided into 2–3 doses or taken as a tea. At therapeutic levels, there are no known side effects or contraindications.

BLACK COHOSH   *Cimicifuga racemosa*

Part used: Rhizome.

Actions: Anti-inflammatory, hypotensive, mild sedative/nervine, antispasmodic.

Therapeutics: Black cohosh was listed in the United States Pharmacopeia from 1820 to 1936 and in the National Formulary from 1936 to 1950. Historically, Eclectic physicians used it for rheumatoid and myalgic pain and a number of modern studies have confirmed black cohosh's anti-inflammatory activity. It is indicated for muscular aches, rheumatoid arthritis and neuralgic pains. It is also a popular herbal remedy for female ailments and its use has been approved in Germany for menopausal disorders and menstrual difficulties. Research shows that it both reduces

LH (lutenizing hormone) and contains isoferulic acid (reduces body temperature) which may account for its ability to reduce hot flashes. An isoflavone in the root binds to estrogen receptors and produces estrogen-like action. Clinical studies have shown that it works as well as estrogens in relieving menopausal symptoms in women after hysterectomies.

Dosage: Follow label instructions for commercial preparations or take ½–1 tsp. of tincture 3 times per day. Do not exceed 4 tsp. per day. Excessive doses can lead to frontal headache, disorientation, nausea, vomiting, impaired circulation and decreased blood pressure. Due to a reported hypotensive effect, caution may also be appropriate for those with low blood pressure. The German Commission E monograph suggests duration of use not to exceed 6 months. Occassional gastrointestinal discomfort has also been reported.

Contraindications: Do not use during pregnancy and lactation.

BOGBEAN   *Menyanthes trifoliata*

Part used: Leaves (gathered in summer after flowering).

Actions: Antirheumatic, digestive stimulant, diuretic.

Therapeutics: Bogbean has a long history as a folk remedy for rheumatism and arthritis. It is a strongly bitter herb that stimulates the secretion of digestive juices and bile flow. It is believed to be particularly effective for rheumatoid arthritis that is accompanied by weakness, weight loss and lack of vitality. Usually, it is combined with other herbs such as black cohosh and celery seed. Celery seed also has a long history in the treatment of rheumatism, arthritis and gout and has been shown to have significant anti-inflammatory action in animal studies. However, do not use celery seed during pregnancy or with kidney inflammation.

Dosage: Use 1–2 tsp. of dried herb and cover with a cup of boiling water. Allow to infuse for 10–15 minutes and drink 3 times a day. For tincture, take ½ to 1 tsp. 3 times a day. For other preparations, follow label instructions.

Contraindications: Do not take bogbean if suffering from diarrhea or colitis. In high doses, gastrointestinal distress is sometimes encountered.

BOSWELLIA (Frankincense) *Boswellia serrata*

Part used: Gum resin.

Actions: Antiarthritic, anti-inflammatory, circulatory stimulant.

Therapeutics: This centuries old herb, commonly known as frankincense, has been used traditionally in India to relieve arthritis discomfort and skin disorders. Now boswellic acid extracts are available which appear to offer even better results. Studies show that boswellia interferes with leukotriene formation by inhibiting lipoxygenase.[49] As we have seen, the leukotriene pathway, which is triggered by the enzyme lipoxygenase, is involved in several inflammatory disorders including Crohn's disease, ulcerative colitis, asthma, hayfever and eczema. Boswellia appears to effectively inhibit the inflammatory process in these disorders and clinical research has also verified the positive effects of

97

boswellia in arthritic patients.[50] Other mechanisms of action in addition to inhibition of inflammatory chemicals include shrinking inflamed tissue by improving blood supply to the affected area, enhancing repair of damaged blood vessels and increasing synovial fluid viscosity in joints. In summary, boswellia has powerful anti-inflammatory effects which have proven helpful in many inflammatory conditions without the side effects associated with most anti-inflammatory and anti-arthritic drugs.

Other Ayurvedic herbs that are combined with boswellia for rheumatoid arthritis include *Commiphora mukul* which is reported to possess powerful anti-inflammatory effects. It's antiarthritic activity was comparable to hydrocortisone and more potent than phenylbutazone[51] and is considered the best medicine for arthritic conditions in India. *Commiphora mukul*, called guggul in India, is distinct from myrrh (*commiphora molmol*) although the two are closely related. The dosage for a standardized extract of 10% gugulipids is 250-500 mg 2-3 times per day. Ashwagandha (*Withania somnifera*) is another herb used in Ayurvedic medicine for rheumatoid arthritis and asthma. It has a steroid like structure and modifies inflammatory leukotrienes to the favorable anti-inflammatory prostaglandin series. It's anti-inflammatory activity has also been compared to hydrocortisone. The suggested dosage is the root powder, 3 grams, 3 times per day or a standardized extract, 500 mg 2-3 times per day.[52] Turmeric is also widely used for arthritis in Ayurvedic medicine and is treated separately in this materia medica.

Dosage: A standard dosage for arthritis is 300-600 mg of standardized 50% boswellic acids, 2-3 times daily. No side effects have been reported.

BUPLEURUM ROOT   *Bupleurum falcatum* and *B. chinensis*
Part used: Root.

Actions: Anti-inflammatory, immune stimulant, hepatoprotective, lowers cholesterol, nephroprotective activity, antitussive, diaphoretic, fever reducing.

Therapeutics: Bupleurum root contains steroid-like molecules known as saikosaponins which have significant anti-inflammatory action. These saikosaponins apparently increase the release of cortisone by the adrenal glands and potentiate its anti-inflammatory effect. This Chinese herb is specifically indicated for chronic inflammatory disorders, especially autoimmune diseases involving the liver or kidneys and for allergies. This herb may be useful on its own as an anti-inflammatory or can be used as an adjunct to steroid therapy to help prevent adrenal gland atrophy. It is also useful in both acute and chronic liver diseases, chemical liver damage and poor liver function. In addition, it is used in cases of gastric ulceration and for acute infections, common cold and chronic cough.

Dosage: 1.5–6 grams of dried root or ¾–2¼ tsp. per day of a 1:2 fluid extract.

Contraindications: Bupleurum root has a sedative effect in some people and can also increase bowel movements and gas, specially in large doses. It can also occasionally cause nausea.

CALENDULA   *Calendula officinalis*

Part used: Flowers.

Actions: Anti-inflammatory, antispasmodic, vulnerary (heals wounds), antiseptic, astringent and detoxifying.

Therapeutics: Calendula is an excellent remedy for red and inflamed skin. It is antiseptic, prevents the spread of infection and speeds up the rate of repair via its granulation-promoting effects. In Europe, calendula is used topically to treat skin and mucous membrane inflammations, slow-healing wounds, leg ulcers, mild burns and sunburn. Internally, calendula exerts valuable anti-inflammatory effects in the digestive system. It is used in the treatment of gastric and duodenal ulcers, gastritis, colitis and diverticulitis. The triterpenoids and flavonoids in it have been linked to its anti-inflammatory activity. Also a cholagogue, it gently stimulates bile flow while soothing irritated mucous membranes throughout the digestive tract (mouth to anus). It has long been considered a detoxifying herb and is used to treat systemic skin disorders such as eczema and acne.

Dosage: For tea, pour a cup of boiling water over 1–2 tsp. of flowers and allow to infuse for 10–15 minutes. Drink 1 cup, 3 times a day. For inflammations of the mucous membranes of the mouth and throat, the still warm tea may be used as a wash or gargle several times a day. Tincture: 1 tsp., 3 times a day. For other commercial preparations, follow label directions. Externally, the tincture can be dabbed on with cotton or salves can be used.

CHAMOMILE   *Matricaria recutita,* formerly *M. chamomilla*

Part used: Flowers.

Actions: Anti-inflammatory, anticatarrhal, antimicrobial, antispasmodic, carminative (expels gas), nervine relaxant and vulnerary (promotes wound healing).

100

Therapeutics: The flavonoid and essential oil components of chamomile possess significant anti-inflammatory and antiallergy activity. Chamomile helps prevent the formation of ulcers and reduces the inflammation in the digestive tract found in gastritis, diverticulitis and colitis. It also helps ease spasms, nervous stomachs and gas and has been used to help ease joint pain associated with arthritis. It has an antispasmodic effect on the body's smooth muscles. The volatile oils in chamomile are believed to decrease histamine release. Externally, its anti-inflammatory effects are also quite strong when used as a steam inhalation for irritated nasal and throat passages and for bronchitis. It is also an excellent remedy for wounds since it is antimicrobial and anti-inflammatory. It soothes the skin and is widely used in Europe for treatment of complaints such as eczema and dry skin. In one study, chamomile was more helpful in speeding the time for skin healing than cortisone. It can help soothe burns, sunburn, diaper rash and even bed sores.

Dosage: Internally, make a tea of 1 tsp. of the dried flowers in a cup of hot water and take 3 times a day. For liquid extracts, take ½ teaspoon 3 times a day or 1–2 teaspoons of tincture in hot water to help evaporate alcohol. For other commercial preparations follow label instructions.

Contraindications: Contact allergies have been reported but are extremely rare. Persons with allergies to pollen such as ragweed may also be allergic to chamomile and may want to avoid its use as an anti-inflammatory. However, Varro Tyler points out that of the 50 reported allergic reactions to chamomiles, only five were attributed to German chamomile, which attests to its relative safety.

Chinese skullcap   *Scutellaria baicalensis*

Part used: Root.

Actions: Anti-inflammatory, antiallergenic, antioxidant.

Therapeutics: Chinese skullcap has been used to treat inflammatory related conditions in China and Japan for centuries. The plants root is rich in flavonoids which give it excellent general anti-inflammatory properties and other specific activities which inhibit hypersensitivity reactions, confirming its traditional use in asthma and allergic dermatitis. It has been shown to inhibit the formation of inflammatory agents such as lipoxygenase and cyclo-oxygenase and to have antihistamine activity. Its ability to limit the bronchoconstriction associated with asthma is believed to be related to its inhibtion of leukotriene production by blocking lipoxygenase and as such may also be useful in other inflammatory conditions associated with elevated leukotrienes such as eczema and inflammatory bowel disease. It also possesses significant antioxidant effects, protecting against free radical damage and decreasing inflammatory reactions.[53]

Dosage: Recommended dosage is 2–6 g of dried root per day or 1–2 tsp. per day of a 1:2 fluid extract.

Devil's claw   *Harpagophytum procumbens*

Part used: Cut, dry tubers.

Actions: Anti-inflammatory, analgesic, digestive stimulant.

Therapeutics: Devil's claw is a South African plant and has been used throughout southern Africa as a treatment for inflammatory diseases, especially arthritis. It has also been used in some hospitals and clinics in Germany and is used as an arthritis treatment in this country, however, opinion is divided on its effectiveness. Some clinical studies have demonstrated encouraging results, finding significant inflammatory relief while others have found it ineffective. In 1962, the active component, harpagoside, was identified, since then one study demonstrated that harpagoside has anti-inflammatory action comparable to phenylbutazone (a potent NSAID). In practice it appears to be effective in easing the symptoms of joint pain. Although clinical studies have not been consistent, it appears to be useful for the treatment of chronic rheumatism, arthritis, gout, myalgia and fibrositis. And even though the evidence is not conclusive, there is enough empirical evidence to warrant further research investigation of this plant and to recommend it as a possible treatment option.

As a bitter herb, devil's claw stimulates gastric secretions and has been effective in treating dyspepsia and stimulating appetite. Many arthritic conditions are associated with poor digestion and malabsorption, so this strong bitter action which stimulates the digestive system may also contribute to the herb's therapeutic value as an anti-inflammatory for arthritis.

Dosage: For a tea, simmer 1 tsp. of dried tuber (root) in 1 cup of water for 10–15 minutes. Drink in small doses throughout the day. For tincture, take 1 tsp. with hot water 3 times a day. For other preparations, take as directed on label.

Contraindications: Don't use with gastric and duodenal ulcers; with gallstones, use only after consultation with a health professional.

DONG QUAI   *Angelica sinensis*

Part used: Root.

Actions: Blood tonic in Chinese herbalism, anti-inflammatory, platelet-activating factor (PAF) inhibitor.

Therapeutics: Although dong quai has an important role in regulating female reproductive disorders, Chinese herbalists also use it to prevent and relieve allergies. Its anti-inflammatory action is linked to its ability to inhibit PAF and to decrease mast cell reactivity and secretion. It is also believed to inhibit the production of antibodies associated with allergic reactions. It relaxes smooth muscles, especially in the trachea, and has active constituents that inhibit the airway spasm associated with asthma.

Dosage: Take the recommended dosage on product labels. For example, a 1:1 extract calls for 10–20 drops, 3 times a day.

EPHEDRA   *Ephedra sinica*

Part used: Stems.

Actions: Antiasthmatic, bronchial dilator, decongestant, expectorant, cardiac stimulant.

Therapeutics: Ephedra is excellent for asthma and respiratory conditions such as congestive sinus conditions. It contains two ephedra alkaloids commonly used in over-the-counter preparations for hay fever and asthma. One is pseudoephedrine, which is used extensively as a decongestant. The other, ephedrine, assists bronchodilation, thereby relieving asthma attacks. In clinical trials, ephedrine alkaloids demonstrated significant anti-inflammatory effects which were believed to be due to prostaglandin inhibition.[54]

However, since ephedra contains ephedrine, it can produce similar side effects, such as increased heart rate, increased blood pressure, anxiety and insomnia, although using the whole plant rather than its active constituent alone probably reduces potential side effects. Ephedrine dosage should not exceed 150 mg in 24 hours in order to avoid side effects such as increased heart rate, high blood pressure, motor disturbances, glaucoma, urinary disturbances, insomnia and nervous behavior.

Ephedra has become a controversial herb recently due to its abuse as a stimulant for weight loss and its inappropriate use in "herbal high" formulations; however, it is an extremely valuable herb when used properly.

Dosage: 1–2g of dried herb divided into 2 to 3 doses or 1 tsp. of dried herb per cup of boiling water, steeped 15 minutes. Drink 2 cups daily. Two g or 1 tsp. of dried herb contains approximately 15–30 mg of ephedrine per cup.

Tincture: 1 tsp. 2–3 times daily. Ephedra is best used in combination with other herbs such as reishi mushroom and siberian ginseng to protect the adrenals since, if used alone for long periods, it can have a weakening effect on the adrenal glands.

Contraindications: The FDA advisory board for over-the-counter drugs has recommended that ephedrine not be taken in cases of high blood pressure, active heart disease, diabetes, thyroid disease, difficulty in urination due to enlarged prostate, glaucoma or if taking an MAO inhibitor or any other prescription drug. These contraindications also apply to ephedra since it contains ephedrine as one of its constituents. In addition, do not take ephedra if you are pregnant or breast-feeding, if you have stimulant sensitivities or if you are taking other over-the-counter antihistamines. If symptoms appear after use and are not relieved in an hour or if they worsen, seek a physician's advice.

If ephedra is contraindicated, use alternative bronchial dilators which do not contain ephedrine alkaloids such as crampbark or black haw. Lobelia is another alternative for bronchial asthma if ephedra is contraindicated since it relaxes the smaller bronchial tube muscles (opening airways), stimulates breathing and promotes expectoration of excess mucus. However, use with caution; may cause nausea and vomiting and is toxic in high doses.

FEVERFEW   *Tanacetum parthenium*

Part used: Leaves.

Action: Migraine preventative, anti-inflammatory.

Therapeutics: Feverfew was used by the ancient Greeks and was even mentioned by Dioscorides as a potent anti-inflammatory. It has been used as an anti-inflammatory to treat fever, arthritis and migraines for centuries. Recent research has verified its effectiveness in the treatment of migraine headaches. However, like other migraine treatments, it is not effective for everyone. Although its mechanism of action is not fully understood, it has been shown to restrict the formation of arachidonic acid by inhibiting the phospholipase pathway and the enzyme cyclooxygenase, preventing formation of inflammatory prostaglandins, thromboxanes and leukotrienes. It is also believed to inhibit

106

degranulation and release of inflammatory chemicals like histamine. As such, it is another anti-inflammatory to consider for
allergies and asthma. It also stabilizes blood platelets and inhibits the release of serotonin from platelets. The overall effect of
these actions is a significant decrease in the inflammatory response. The chemical serotonin is widely believed to be the
primary trigger for migraines, thus the inhibition of its release
probably accounts for the reduction in severity, duration and
frequency of migraines. The inhibition of the release of inflammatory chemicals from white blood cells in inflamed joints
and skin may also account for its use in arthritis.

The active ingredient believed to be responsible for these
actions is parthenolide, however, parthenolide is not found in
all varieties of feverfew. For this reason it has been recommended that the use of feverfew be limited to standardized
preparations stating the level of parthenolides present. Canadian
regulations have adopted a 0.2 percent parthenolide content as
the minimum standard for products and specifically recommend
a daily dosage of 125 mg for the treatment and prevention of
migraines. This equals about 250 mcg of parthenolide daily.
However, some herbalists report good results using freeze dried
leaf preparations and whole plant tinctures. The use of this herb
is best for long-term preventive treatment and not for acute
care of migraines. In addition, approximately 4–6 weeks of con-
tinuous administration is required before a positive response is
noted, although this varies among individuals.

Dosage: For migraine prevention, the daily dose of freeze-dried
leaves is 125 mg of .2 percent parthenolide content. Some practitioners recommend higher dosages for the treatment of rheu-

matoid arthritis than those used in migraine prevention. For rheumatoid arthritis and other inflammatory conditions such as allergies/asthma, the recommendation is 250 (.2%) milligrams daily. For whole plant tinctures, follow product recommendations.

Contraindications: Do not use during pregnancy or lactation and use caution if taking warfarin or other blood-thinning drugs. Do not give to children under age 12. Allergic contact dermatitis has been reported but it is rare. Occasional mouth sores and ulcers have been reported by individuals chewing the fresh leaves, but they disappear after discontinuing use. No major adverse effects have been reported and it appears to be extremely well tolerated.

GINGER   *Zingiber officinale*

Part used: Rhizome.

Actions: Anti-inflammatory, digestive stimulant, carminative (eliminates intestinal gas), antinausea/antivomiting, circulatory stimulant.

Therapeutics: In China, ginger has been used to treat numerous conditions, including rheumatism, for thousands of years. The ayurvedic system of herbal medicine also uses ginger in the treatment of inflammatory joint diseases, including arthritis. In terms of its anti-inflammatory effects, ginger's antioxidant effects are important, plus it inhibits the formation of thromboxanes and leukotrienes, which are potent inflammatory chemicals. It makes platelets less "sticky" or less likely to aggregate by inhib-

iting the action of thromboxane. Fresh ginger also contains protein-digesting enzymes (proteases), which may have plant
protease anti-inflammatory actions similar to bromelain and papain. As such, in cases like rheumatoid arthritis, it may be more
effective than dry preparations. Studies indicate its usefulness
for rheumatoid arthritis, osteoarthritis and muscular pain. Research using powdered ginger for arthritis patients showed that
more than 75 percent experienced pain and swelling relief.
When used for muscular discomfort, all the patients experienced
relief in pain or swelling. The recommended dosage was
500–1,000 mg per day, however, many patients took 3–4 times
this amount. Plus, the patients taking higher doses reported
quicker and better relief. None of the patients reported any
adverse effects during the time they took the ginger, which
ranged from 3 months to 2.5 years.[55]

This plant also possesses digestive system actions relieving
gas and spasms and is a classic tonic for the digestive system;
it also has antinausea actions.

Dosage: ½ to 1 tsp. of dried root, divided into 2–3 portions is
an average daily dose. A dosage of equivalent fresh ginger root
would be approximately a ½-inch slice of fresh ginger root as
part of the diet or juiced. Although most of the studies have
used powdered dry ginger root, fresh ginger root or ginger root
extracts or tinctures may provide even better results since they
contain higher levels of gingerol. For other preparations, such as
extracts or tinctures, use as directed on the label. It should be
noted that the daily doses employed in the reports for arthritis,
osteoarthritis, and muscular pain varied from 3–7 grams powdered
root daily and in India the average daily dose is 8–10 grams.

Contraindications: Although there does not appear to be any toxicity associated with the use of ginger, the German Commission E monograph warns those with gallbladder disease to use it only after consulting with a physician. Nor should it be used for morning sickness in pregnancy unless supervised by a physician.

GINKGO   *Ginkgo biloba*

Part used: Leaf.

Actions: Circulatory tonic, antioxidant, anti-inflammatory (PAF inhibitor), bronchodilator, cerebrovascular tonic.

Therapeutics: Ginkgo is the oldest living tree species in the world and its medicinal use can be traced back almost 5,000 years in Chinese medicine. In an early Chinese materia medica the leaves were recommended for asthma as well as memory loss. Today, ginkgo is highly valued for these and other reasons. Ginkgo is very useful for people with allergies and asthma due to its ability to inhibit platelet-activating factor (PAF). It is also high in flavonoids and has profound membrane-stabilizing, free radical scavenger and antioxidant effects which are very helpful in addressing inflammation. Other applications or uses include early stages of Alzheimer's disease, varicose veins, senility, ringing in the ear, eczema, multiple sclerosis, poor circulation to the extremities and atherosclerosis, among others.

Dosage: Nearly all the studies with ginkgo have been done on standardized extracts. Thus, for predictable results the suggested dosage is 80–160 mg of 24-percent flavone glycosides, in three divided doses. A treatment period of approximately 4–6 weeks is usually required before effective responses are seen. Whole plant extracts may be as effective as the standardized extracts, but no comparison studies are available. Follow dosage recommendations on labels for other preparations. Some herbalists recommend that ginkgo be used for a minimum of three months to be truly beneficial.

Contraindications: There are no known toxicities associated with the herb and it appears safe for long-term use and for use by pregnant or lactating women at recommended dosages. Some adverse effects have been anecdotally reported when taken with aspirin or blood thinning courmarins. Thus, use with anticoagulant medications should be closely monitored. Mild side effects, although rare, include gastrointestinal upset, and, in people with poor blood flow to the brain, mild headaches during initial use.

GOLDENROD   *Solidago* spp.

Part used: Herb/flowers.

Actions: Anticatarrhal, anti-inflammatory, mucous membrane antiseptic, astringent, diuretic.

Therapeutics: Goldenrod is a gentle herb with no known toxicity and it has been used traditionally for hay fever and allergies, helping to prevent constant outflow or drainage from sinuses. It contains tannins, saponins, flavonoids and phenolic glycosides, including leiocarposide, which has been found to have anti-inflammatory and analgesic actions for both the upper respiratory tract and urinary tract. Leiocarposide is converted to salicylic acid in the intestinal tract, so this probably accounts for its anti-inflammatory action. Goldenrod is specifically indicated in cases of chronic nasal congestion.

Dosage: Take 1 cup tea, 2 times daily. For acute conditions, drink 1 cup every 3–4 hours with the last dose at least 2 hours before bed to prevent nighttime urination urge. Prepare by pouring 1 cup boiling water over 2 tsp. herb/flowers. Steep for 15 minutes. Strain and drink. In tincture form, use as directed on label. For hay fever, start taking a few weeks before hay fever season, as well as throughout the season.

GUAIACUM   *Guaiacum officinale*

Part used: Heartwood.

Actions: Anti-inflammatory, antirheumatic, diuretic (when used cold), laxative, diaphoretic (when used hot).

Therapeutics: The heartwood of this tree is rich in resinous acids and saponins. It is primarily used for rheumatoid arthritis and chronic rheumatism due to its potent anti-inflammatory action. It can be combined effectively with bogbean, meadowsweet or celery seed. In addition, some also find it beneficial for osteoarthritis. It has also been used for the treatment of gout, relieving pain and inflammation in between attacks and reducing the frequency of attacks. As a reputed circulatory stimulant it reduces inflammatory responses by improving circulation to the affected tissues.

Dosage: Simmer 1 tsp. of the wood chips in 12 oz. of water, simmer for 15 minutes. Drink ⅓ cup, 3–4 times daily.

Contraindications: Guaiacum has a high content of resins, thus caution should be used in people with gastritis, peptic ulcers or those with allergic hypersensitivities.

HAWTHORN *Crataegus oxycantha*

Part used: Fruit, leaves and flower.

Actions: Heart tonic, antioxidant, supportive antiallergenic.

Therapeutics: Although best known for its primary action as a heart tonic, strengthening heart muscle force of contraction and improving blood flow, hawthorn also possesses antihistamine and antioxidant activity. Hawthorn blocks conversion of histadine to histamine. It is high in flavonoids, including proanthocyanidins and quercetin, making it an effective antioxidant counteracting the damaging effects of free radicals involved in inflammatory conditions.

Dosage: Tea: Pour one cup of boiling water over 2 tsp. of berries and leaves and allow to infuse for 15–20 minutes. Strain and drink 3 times per day. Tincture: Take 1 tsp. 3 times a day. For other preparations, follow recommendations on product labels.

LICORICE *Glycyrrhiza glabra*

Part used: Root.

Actions: Anti-inflammatory, antiallergenic, expectorant, demulcent, antispasmodic, adaptogenic, mild laxative.

Therapeutics: Licorice is one of the most biologically active herbs known. It has extensive therapeutic use worldwide and has been researched extensively. It has broad anti-inflammatory activity due to its steroid-like, cortisol-enhancing effects similar to hydrocortisone and other corticosteroid hormones. In addition, it helps block the release of histamine and serotonin from mast cells and stabilizes mast cell membranes, making it less likely to spill out inflammatory chemicals. Licorice also inhibits the enzyme phospholipase, which is responsible for releasing arachidonic acid, leading to leukotriene formation and inflammatory prostaglandins. Virtually any inflammatory condition can be reduced by licorice and it is a key herb for arthritis, allergies and asthma. Other possible applications include eczema, IBD, heartburn, peptic ulcers, chronic hepatitis, cirrhosis, and PMS.

Dosage: Recommended adult dosage is 1 tsp. of tincture 3 times a day or ½ tsp. of fluid extract, 3 times a day. Decoction tea: 1 tsp. root per cup water (start with a little extra water since some will evaporate while simmering); simmer 10–15 minutes. Take 1 cup 3 times daily.

Contraindications: The duration of use suggested in the German Commission E Monograph is 4–6 weeks, without consulting a physician. Licorice root taken in excessive amounts can result in potassium loss, sodium retention and hypertension. However, the sensitivity to these side effects varies among individuals, and some herbalists believe that its potential negative side effects have been greatly exaggerated. Many herbalists believe that its potential side effects can be counteracted by a high-potassium, low-sodium diet. In order to prevent potential side effects, especially over an extended period of time, a multi mineral supplement with potassium is strongly advised along with instituting a high-potassium, e.g., bananas, potatoes, dried apricots, orange juice and other potassium-rich fruits and vegetables, low-sodium diet during the duration of use. Do not use in high blood pressure, pregnancy, liver cirrhosis, low potassium, edema or history of heart or kidney problems, or when taking potassium-depleting diuretics.

LOBELIA   *Lobelia inflata*

Part used: Herb.

Actions: Antispasmodic, bronchial dilator, expectorant, respiratory stimulant and emetic.

Therapeutics: Lobelia is a useful herb for asthma and chronic bronchitis. It reduces secretions while promoting expectoration and helps relax bronchial muscles; thus, spasmodic asthma seems to respond well to it.

Dosage: The adult dosage of dried aerial parts, using a 1:5 tincture is .3 ml–1 ml or 10–20 drops, 3 times a day. Start at low end of dosage range and work upwards as needed. Dried plant tinctures are less potent since the alkaloids and glycosides are diminished by drying, so do not use fresh plant tinctures without the guidance of a skilled practitioner and avoid capsules.

Contraindications: Use caution when taking this herb as it can cause dose-dependent cardioactivity in large doses. Lobelia should not be taken during pregnancy, by nursing mothers or by persons with hyperactive upper GI systems. Nausea and vomiting can occur in high doses or in sensitive people.

MEADOWSWEET   *Filipendula ulmaria*

Part used: Herb.

Actions: Anti-inflammatory, antiacid, astringent, diuretic.

Therapeutics: Meadowsweet contains salicylates, which are aspirin-like substances, and as such help reduce inflammation and provide pain relief. It is used in inflammatory conditions, particularly arthritis. In addition, it is an excellent digestive remedy which protects and soothes the digestive tract mucous membranes, reducing excess acidity. It is used for the treatment of duodenal and gastric ulcers (especially for alcohol and NSAID-induced ulcers) and gastritis. Although salicylates have been associated with stomach bleeding, meadowsweet contains tannins, mucilage and other constituents which assist mucosal healing and it is not metabolized the same way as aspirin. Thus, it does not cause the same problems that aspirin can in the stomach.

Combined with chamomile and marshmallow it is very soothing to a range of digestive problems. For arthritis it is helpful combined with black cohosh, willow bark and celery seed.

Dosage: 1 cup of boiling water to 1–2 tsp. of dried herb; infuse for 10–15 minutes. Drink 1 cup, 3 times daily, or as needed. For tinctures, take ½–1 teaspoon, 3 times a day. For other preparations, follow label instructions.

Contraindications: Although there have been no reported cases in the literature it may be appropriate for those with salicylate hypersensitivities and those taking prescription drugs that carry aspirin warnings to exercise caution.

NETTLE   *Urtica dioica*

Part used: Dried leaves.

Actions: Mild diuretic, alterative (tonic), astringent, anti-allergenic.

Therapeutics: Nettle is an excellent cleansing, detoxifying herb which possesses a mild diuretic action. It has been found helpful in eczema, arthritic conditions and gout. It is also antiallergenic and is useful in the treatment of allergic conditions such as hay fever and asthma.

Dosage: The recommended dosage is 450 mg, 2–3 times daily of freeze-dried nettle herb, especially for allergies. Alternatively, other preparations are also recommended. Take 40–60 drops of fresh leaf extract 3 times daily or take ½–1 tsp. of tincture diluted in 1 cup of hot water, 3 times a day. To prepare a tea, pour 1 cup boiling water over 2 tsp. of herb and steep for 15 minutes. Strain and drink 3 cups per day. For fresh juice, take 1–2 tsp., 3 times a day. For liquid extracts take ½–1 tsp., 3 times daily. For seasonal allergies, it is advisable to start taking nettle one month before and throughout allergy season. Discontinue one month after allergy season has ended.

117

SARSAPARILLA   *Smilax officinalis*

Part used: Root and rhizome.

Actions: Anti-inflammatory, antirheumatic, diuretic, diaphoretic, alterative.

Therapeutics: Sarsaparilla has been used throughout the world, in many different cultures, for similar conditions, namely gout, arthritis, psoriasis, eczema and ulcerative colitis. It contains saponins which bind to bacterial endotoxins in the intestines and promote their excretion. It may also work as an anti-inflammatory by enhancing endogenous steroid levels. Sarsaparilla has a general tonic effect on the whole body.

  Clinical experience with sarsaparilla extracts have produced favorable results in psoriasis where out of 92 patients, 62 percent experienced great improvement and another 18 percent experienced total clearance of symptoms.[56]

Dosage: For a decoction tea, use 1–2 tsp. of the root in 1 cup of water and bring to a boil, simmering for 10–15 minutes. Drink 1 cup, 3 times daily. For liquid extracts, take ½–1 tsp. 3 times a day. For other types of preparation, take as directed on label.

SKUNK CABBAGE   *Symplocarpus foetidus*

Part used: Root.

Actions: Expectorant, respiratory sedative, antispasmodic.

Therapeutics: This herb was a favorite of Native Americans and was in the official USP (United States Pharmacopoeia) from

1820–82 as an antispasmodic. It is a gentle but effective expectorant, a strong antispasmodic on respiratory passages and a bronchial relaxant helping to ease persistent coughs.

Dosage: Use in minute dosages only since it is high in volatile oils and can be irritating. Do not use fresh plant tincture. It is best used in a formula with other asthma herbs and under the direction of a medical herbalist or naturopath. The recommended daily tincture dosage is ¼ th tsp. or 20 drops, 3 times a day. Small amounts of chili pepper are often used with skunk cabbage, along with lobelia. Chili pepper desensitizes respiratory mucosa to a variety of mechanical and chemical irritants.

Contraindications: Individuals with a history of kidney stones should use this herb cautiously due to its high oxalate content.

TURMERIC   *Curcuma longa*

Part used: Yellow pigment (curcumin) or rhizome.

Actions: Anti-inflammatory, antioxidant, antiplatelet aggregator, stimulates bile secretion.

Therapeutics: Tumeric has been used as a spice and medicine for thousands of years. It was mentioned in an Assyrian herbal dating from 600 BC and Dioscorides also referred to it. Today, modern scientific studies have confirmed a range of clinical actions. It possesses a unique combination of properties such as anti-inflammatory, antioxidant, digestive, antiplatelet, cholesterol lowering and possible anticancer effects. In fact, curcumin which is the yellow pigment in turmeric may be one of nature's most potent anti-inflammatories. Its direct anti-inflammatory effects include inhibition of the formation of leukotrienes, inhibition of platelet aggregation, reduction of swelling by promoting the breakdown of fibrin, inhibition of the release of other inflammatory chemicals by white blood cells and stabilization of the cell membranes of lysosomes so they don't spill their inflammatory chemicals as easily. In addition to these direct inflammatory actions, curcumin also appears to increase the activity of the body's anti-inflammatory mechanisms.[57] Both animal studies and clinical human trials have demonstrated that curcumin's powerful anti-inflammatory action is just as strong as phenylbutazone but without any side effects at recommended dosages. However, curcumin does not have any direct pain-relieving actions.

Curcumin is also a powerful antioxidant, and preliminary research has shown protective effects against the development of cancer. Possible applications, among others, include the treatment of inflammatory conditions such as rheumatoid arthritis, IBD, asthma, allergies and eczema.

Dosage: An effective anti-inflammatory response requires a dosage of 400–600 mg 3 times a day of curcumin. To get a similar amount by consuming turmeric would require 8,000 to 60,000 mg, so using curcumin in supplement form is usually recommended instead. Curcumin, often combined with bromelain to help enhance its absorption, is best taken before meals or between meals. However, some herbalists report results simply using powdered turmeric at a dose of 4 tsp. a day. A tsp. of powdered turmeric can be mixed with water or milk (preferably rice or soy) to a slurry and drunk 4 times per day. A tsp. of

120

lecithin can also be added to enhance absorption. Alternatively mix 1 tsp. of turmeric in 1 cup of vanilla rice or soy milk and simmer gently (do not boil) for 3-5 mintues. Three cardomom pods can also be added if desired. Allow to cool and just before drinking add 1 tsp. of flaxseed oil (optional). Sweetner (honey or maple syrup) can also be added to taste or try serving with a little cinnamon sprinkled on top. It makes an excellent bedtime drink.

Contraindications: Curcumin is contraindicated for those with gallstones or an obstructed biliary tract unless used under a physician's supervision. Persons taking antiplatelet drugs should not take high doses.

TYLOPHORA   *Tylophora asthmatica*

Part used: Leaves

Actions: Antiasthmatic, antispasmodic, antihistamine.

Therapeutics: Tylophora is a popular asthma and respiratory herb in ayurvedic herbal medicine. It offers significant relief for the symptoms of hay fever and asthma. It appears to inhibit mast cell degranulation, preventing the release of inflammatory chemicals, and it improves respiratory function.

Dosage: The dose is 200 mg of the powdered leaf 2 times daily. For powdered extracts, the dose is 40 mg daily. For a 1:5 tincture take 40–80 drops 2 times a day.

Contradications: Do not exceed the recommended dosages since toxicity and side effects like nausea, vomiting and dry mouth

121

can occur at high doses. Tylophora, like ephedra, contains alkaloids, thus long-term use is probably not advised. It is recommended that this herb be taken only under the supervision of a skilled practitioner.

WILD YAM   *Dioscorea villosa*

Part used: Root.

Actions: Anti-inflammatory, antirheumatic, antispasmodic, bile stimulant, expectorant, diuretic, increases sweating.

Therapeutics: Wild yam contains steroidal saponins such as diosgenin, which are believed to inhibit prostaglandins that cause inflammation. It is very useful in rheumatoid arthritis formulas due to its combined anti-inflammatory and antispasmodic actions, which reduce inflammation, pain and relax stiff muscles. It is helpful combined with black cohosh and may be used in anti-inflammatory formulas as a licorice substitute for hypertensive individuals. Its combined anti-inflammatory and antispasmodic effects are also specific for inflammation of the bowel and stomach. As such, it is particularly useful for irritable bowel syndrome (IBS), ulcerative colitis, diverticulitis, cramping, intestinal colic and liver and gallbladder inflammation. In addition, it has also been used for painful uterine contractions during menstruation.

Dosage: For a decoction tea, place 1–2 tsp. of root in 1 cup of water and bring to a boil, then simmer for 10–15 minutes. Drink 1 cup, 3 times a day. For tinctures take ½–1 tsp., 3 times daily. For other preparations, such as fluid extracts, follow product label directions.

WILLOW BARK   *Salix* spp. (especially *purpurea* and *fragilis*)

Part used: Bark.

Actions: Anti-inflammatory, reduces muscle aches and pains, analgesic, astringent.

Therapeutics: Willow is considered a "natural aspirin" and is the classic anti-inflammatory herb. It contains salicylates which inhibit the formation of prostaglandins and the actions of white blood cells that are involved in inflammation. Willow bark is indicated for rheumatic and arthritic disorders as well as pain caused by inflammation. Willow, as well as all salicylate-rich herbs, however, takes about 6–10 hours to achieve a therapeutically adequate and steady blood level, so it is not very effective for acute inflammatory use. It is, however, extremely effective for chronic pain and inflammation such as chronic arthritic pain or chronic joint aches and does not directly irritate the stomach lining like aspirin does. It is optimally effective after taking for at least 72 hours or 3 days. Unlike aspirin, willow does not thin the blood, so do not rely on it for this action.

Dosage: For a decoction tea, place 1 tsp. of root in 1 cup of water and bring to a boil, then simmer for 10–15 minutes. Drink 1 cup, 3 times a day. For tinctures take 1–2 tsp., 3 times daily. For other preparations, such as fluid extracts, capsules or tablets, follow label directions.

Contraindications: Although there are no reported cases in the literature it may be appropriate for those with salicylate hypersensitivities and those taking prescription drugs that carry aspirin warnings to exercise caution. Even though salicylate side effects are unlikely, some practitioners also caution against its use in high fever conditions by children under age 15 due to the possibility of Reye's syndrome. Although there is a well known tendency for aspirin to cause gastric bleeding, there are no reports of this effect in salicin containing herbs. However, willow does produce salicylic acid in the body which blocks the enzyme cycloxygenase. This enzyme inhibits not only inflammatory prostaglandins but also prostacyclin which is considered to be a protective prostaglandin in the mucus membranes of the stomach and G.I. tract. Thus, significant quantities used long term could potentially lead to gastrointestional irritation.

YUCCA   *Yucca* spp.

Part used: Root.

Actions: Anti-inflammatory, antirheumatic, laxative.

Therapeutics: Yucca root contains steroidal saponins which are believed to produce cortisone-like activity or which may act as precursors for the body's own conversion to cortisone. These constituents may explain its exceptional traditional anti-inflammatory use. Yucca has been used by traditional peoples of both North and South America for relief of rheumatic pain. It is a very useful anti-inflammatory for the treatment of both osteo and rheumatoid arthritis.[58] Digestive demulcents can be added when taking yucca if the saponins cause an upset stomach. Yucca combined with chaparral is a traditional southwestern herbal remedy for arthritis. Chaparral is a potent antioxidant, however, it is contraindicated for those who have had or may have had liver disease and use should be discontinued if nausea, fever, fatigue or jaundice occur. A combined yucca and chapparral mixture is available from Tieraona's Herbals. (See Resources.) Yucca can also be combined with yerba mansa for arthritis relief. Yerba mansa is another widely used southwestern herbal remedy for arthritis and has reported aspirin-like anti-inflammatory effects.

Dosage: Take as directed on product labels. To prepare your own: chop about 4 oz, of the dry inner root (without bark) into small pieces (approximately 1 cup) and place it in a crock pot with 48 oz. (6 cups) of water. Set on the lowest setting with lid on and cook for about 1½–2 days, watching carefully so that about 3–4 inches are left in bottom. Strain out the root and continue to cook with lid off for about 12 hours until all that is left is about 2 inches of black syrup on the bottom of the crock pot. Take this out, bottle, and keep refrigerated. Suggested dosage is about 10 drops, 3 times daily. Alternatively, boil approximately ⅓ cup (¼ oz.) of chopped dry inner root in 2 cups of water for 15 minutes. Strain and drink ½ cup, 4 times a day.

Contraindications: In large amounts intestinal irritation can occur leading to a laxative effect and intestinal cramping. Thus, it is contraindicated in pregnancy and colitis. Long term use should also be avoided due to a potential reduction in absorption of fat-soluable vitamins.

Conclusions

An effective immune system and inflammatory response are crucial for health. If our inflammatory response is inadequate, we aren't able to fend off infections and illness and aren't able to effectively repair and replace cells destroyed by normal wear and tear. However, if our inflammatory system is excessive and overactive or hyperreactive, it can damage healthy tissues and lead to chronic inflammatory diseases. For those who suffer from chronic inflammatory diseases, there are natural approaches that can help the body restore balance and offer relief without causing additional problems.

To balance the inflammatory response, eat a well-balanced diet with lots of colorful organic fruits and vegetables and consume cold-water fatty fish. Avoid dietary animal fats which can increase inflammation and avoid hydrogenated oils with transfatty acids. Take high-quality essential fatty acids like EPA-rich fish oil or flaxseed oil and avoid drugs and chemicals that can increase sensitivity to inflammation. Drink sufficient quantities of water to assist in detoxification and optimize digestion with digestive enzymes or herbal bitters. In addition, take the dietary supplements discussed such as nutrients and herbs that are natural anti-inflammatories and antioxidants. Finally, consider the herbs indicated for the specific system or condition involved in addition to general circulatory, eliminative and liver herbs.

Positive changes in diet, avoidance of environmental toxins and food additives, together with the use of specific herbs and nutrients mentioned throughout this book can help to dramatically reduce inflammation, pain and swelling. Like Manuel Cordova, Amazon jungle healer, I believe that "since man is a product of nature . . . a cure for all of his ills will be found in nature and those cures are natural . . . and not miraculous at all."[59] Green blessings on your path to health and wellness.

Appendix:
Supplemental Herb List

Agrimony herb	*Agrimonia eupatorium*
Alfalfa leaf	*Medicago sativa*
Anise seed	*Pimpinella anisum*
Ashwagandha root	*Withania somnifera*
Aspen/Cottonwood bark	*Populus* spp.
Astragalus root	*Astragalus membranaceus*
Barberry	*Berberis vulgaris*
Bayberry bark	*Myrica cerifera*
Birch bark	*Betula* spp.
Black haw root	*Viburnum prunifolium*
Blue Cohosh root	*Caulophyllum thalictroides*
Burdock root	*Articum lappa*
Canadian fleabane flowering herb	*Erigeron canadensis*
Celery Seed	*Apium graveolens*
Chaparral leaf	*Larrea tridentata*
Chinese Wolfberry root bark	*Lycium chinense*
Cinnamon bark	*Cinnomomum* spp.
Cleavers herb	*Galium aparine*
Coltsfoot flower/leaf	*Tussilago farfara*
Comfrey leaf	*Symphytum officinale* (Caution: Not for internal use)

129

Commiphora mukul (Guggul resin)   *Commiphora mukul*
Corn silk   *Zea mays*
Cramp bark   *Viburnum opulus*
Cranesbill rhizome   *Geranium maculatum*
Dandelion root/leaf   *Taraxacum officinale*
Echinacea root   *Echinacea* spp.
Elder flower/berry   *Sambucus nigra*
Elecampagne root   *Inula helenium*
Eyebright herb   *Euphrasia officinalis*
Fennel seed   *Foeniculum vulgare*
Fenugreek seed   *Trigonella foenum-graecum*
Gentian root   *Gentiana lutea*
Goldenseal root   *Hydrastis canadensis*
Gotu Kola leaf/root   *Centella asiatica*
Grindelia buds/flowers   *Grindelia camporum*
Horse Chestnut   *Aesculus hippocastanum*
Horsetail herb   *Equisetum arvense*
Kava kava root   *Piper methysticum*
Lady's mantle leaf   *Alchemilla vulgaris* or *mollies*
Lavender flowering herb   *Lavandula officinalis*
Lemon balm leaf   *Melissa officinalis*
Linden flowers   *Tilia* spp.
Marshmallow root   *Althaea officinalis*
Milk thistle seed   *Silybum marianum*
Mullein leaf   *Verbascum thapsus*
Oat seed   *Avena sativum*
Oregon Grape root   *Berberis aquifolium*
Oxeye daisy   *Chrysanthemum oxycanthum*
Passion flower herb   *Passiflora incarnata*
Peppermint leaf   *Mentha piperita*
Plantain leaf   *Plantago major*
Pleurisy root   *Asclepias tuberosa*
Poke root   *Phytolacca americana* (Caution: For Professional Use Only)

Prickly ash bark	*Zanthoxylum americanum*
Raspberry leaf	*Rubus idaeus*
Red clover flower	*Trifolium pratense*
Red root	*Ceanothus* spp.
Rehmannia root	*Rehmannia glutinosa*
Reishi mushroom	*Ganoderma lucidum*
Sage leaf	*Salvia officinalis*
Schizandra berry	*Schinzandra chinensis*
Shephard's purse herb	*Capsella bursa-pastoris*
Shitake mushroom	*Lentinula erodes*
Siberian ginseng root	*Eleutherococcus senticosus*
Skullcap herb	*Scutellaria laterifolia*
Slippery Elm bark	*Ulmus fulva* or *rubra*
St. John's Wort flower/herb	*Hypericum perforatum*
Uva Ursi or Bearberry leaf	*Arctostaphylos uva-ursi*
Wild indigo root	*Baptisia tinctoria*
Wintergreen	*Gaultheria procumbens*
Witch Hazel	*Hamamelis virginana*
Wormwood leaf	*Artemiaia absinthum*
Yarrow flower	*Achillea millefolium*
Yellow dock root	*Rumex crispus*
Yerba mansa root	*Anemopsis californica*
Yerba santa leaf	*Eriodictyon* spp.

References

1. Mills, Simon, *The Essential Book of Herbal Medicine*, London, Penguin Books, Ltd., 1991, p. 62.
2. Pizzorno, Joseph E., N.D., and Murray, Michael T., N.D., *A Text book of Natural Medicine*, Rocklin, CA, Prima Publishing, 1994, section IV:BwlTox-1.
3. Mitchell, William, N.D., Lecture on *Alzheimer's*, Pacific NW Herbal Symposium, May 1997, Wilsonville, Oregon.
4. Stansbury, Jill E., N.D., *Herbal Anti-inflammatories: New Research in Pain Management*, Official Proceedings, Medicines from the Earth—Protocols for Botanical Healing, June 1–3, 1996, Blue Ridge Assembly, North Carolina, p. 131.
5. Marieb, Elaine, *Human Anatomy and Physiology*, New York, The Benjamin/Cummings Publishing Company, 1995, pp. 595, 709.
6. Stansbury, p. 127.
7. Ibid, p. 132; Dharmananda, Subhuti, "Chinese Medical Views and Treatments of Allergy," In: *The Protocol Journal of Botanical Medicine*, Vol. 1, No. 2, Autumn 1995; p. 70.
8. Stansbury, p. 134; see also, Burgess, Nick, *Osteoarthritis: Protocols for Effective Botanical Treatment*, in Official Proceedings of the Southwest Conference on Botanical Medicine, April 12–13, 1997, Tempe, Arizona, p. 19.
9. Stansbury, p. 128, 134; see also, Burgess, p. 19, van Loon, Isis M., N.D., "The Golden Root: Clinical Applications of Scutellaria bai-

calensis GEORGI Flavonoids as Modulators of the Inflammatory Response," *Alternative Medicine Review*, Vol. 2, Number 6: 472–480, Dec. 1997; Yoshimoto, T., et al., "Flavonoids: potent inhibitors of arachidonate 5-lipoxygenase," *Biochem Biophys Res Commun*, 116:612, 1983; Yoshimoto, T., et. al., "Arachidonate 5-lipoxygenase and its new inhibitors," *J Allergy Clin Immunol*, 74: 349, 1984.

10. Nogammi Mari, et al., "Studies on Ganoderma lucindum I-VII Anti-allergic effects," *Yagaku*, pp. 594-604, 1986; Willard, Terry, Ph. D., "Asthma & Allergies—Multi-factorial Problems," in *Official Proceedings of the Southwest Conference on Botanical Medicine*, April 20-21, 1996, Tempe, Arizona, p. 117; Holmes, Peter, *Jade Remedies: A Chinese Herbal Reference for the West*, Snow Lotus Press, Boulder, CO, 1997, pp. 554-556.

11. Stansbury, p. 133.

12. Isselbacher, Kurt J., et al., *Harrison's Principles of Internal Medicine*, New York, McGraw-Hill, Inc., 1994, p. 1552.

13. Murray, Michael and Pizzorno, Joseph, *Encyclopedia of Natural Medicine*, Rocklin, CA, Prima Publishing, 1991, pp. 71–72.

14. Pizzorno, Joe, N.D., *Total Wellness*, Rocklin, CA, Prima Publishing, 1996, pp. 167–168.

15. Ibid.

16. Ibid., p. 171.

17. Maseri, A., "Inflammation, atherosclerosis, and ischemic events— exploring the hidden side of the moon," *The New England Journal of Medicine*, 336(14): 1014–1016, 1997.

18. Fisher, M., et al., "Effects of dietary fish oil supplementation on polymorphonuclear leukocyte inflammatory potential," *Inflammation*, 10(4): 387–392, 1986.

19. Ridker, P.M., et al., "Inflammation, aspirin, and the risk of cardio-vascular disease," *New England Journal of Medicine*, 336(14): 973–979, 1997.

20. Murray, Michael, N.D., *Arthritis—How You Can Benefit from Diet, Vitamins, Minerals, Herbs, Exercise and Other Natural Methods*, Rocklin CA, Prima Publishing, 1994, p. 71.

21. Murray, Michael, N.D., "The natural approach to rheumatoid ar-

thritis," *The American Journal of Natural Medicine,* Vol 3: 15–16, Jan./ Feb. 1996.

22. Murray, Michael, N.D., "Essential Fatty Acid Supplementation," in *Encyclopedia of Nutritional Supplements,* Rocklin, CA, Prima Publishing, 1996, pp. 252–253.

23. Mitchell, William, N.D., "Allergies: Immediate-type Hypersensitivity," *The Protocol Journal of Botanical Medicine,* Vol. 1, Number 2, Autumn 1995, pp. 63–67.

24. Murray, "The natural approach to rheumatoid arthritis," pp. 15–16.

25. Gabor, M., "Pharmacologic effects of flavonoids on blood vessels," *Angiologica,* 9:355–374, 1972; Amella M., et al., "Inhibition of mast cell histamine release by flavonoids and bioflavonoids," *Planta Medica,* 51: 16–20, 1985; Bennet, J.P., et. al., "Inhibitory effects of natural flavonoids on secretion from mast cells and neutrophils," *Arzneim-Forsh. Drugs Res,* 31:433, 1981; Yoshimoto, T., et al., "Flavonoids: potent inhibitors of arachidonate 5-lipoxygenase," p. 612; Yoshimoto, T., et al., "Arachidonate 5-lipoxygenase and its new inhibitors," pg. 349.

26. Gabor, Miklos and Razga, *Acta Physiol. Hungary,* 77:197–207, 1991.

27. Innerfield, I., *Enzymes in Clinical Medicine,* New York, McGraw Hill, 1960. Horger, I., "Enzyme therapy in multiple rheumatic diseases," *Therapiewoche,* 33:39948–57, 1983; Ransberger K., "Enzyme treatment of immune complex diseases," *Arthritis Rheuma,* 8:1609, 1986.

28. Gordon, Garry, M.D., D.O., "Aspirin vs. Enzymes," *The Doctor's Prescription for Healthy Living,* Vol. 2, Number 3:10–11, 1998.

29. Deitrick, R.E., "Oral proteolytic enzymes in the treatment of athletic injuries: a double-blind study," *The Pennsylvania Medical Journal,* 68(10):35–37, 1965.

30. Oelgoeetz, A.W., "The treatment of food allergy and indigestion of pancreatic origin with pancreatic enzymes," *Am J Dig Dis Nutr,* 2:422–6, 1935.

31. Tarayre, J.P. and Lauressergues, H., "Advantages of a combination of proteolytic enzymes, flavonoids and ascorbic acid in comparison with nonsteroidal anti-inflammatory agents," *Arzheim Forsch,* 27:1144–9, 1977.

32. Smith, J.M., "Adverse reactions to food and drug additives," *Eur J Clin Nutr*, 45:17–21, 1991.

33. Murray, Michael, N.D., *Natural Alternatives to Over-the-Counter and Prescription Drugs*, New York, William Morrow and Company, Inc., 1994, pp. 68–69.

34. Bingham, R., et al., "Yucca plant saponin in the management of arthritis," *J Appl Nutr*, 27:45–50, 1975.

35. Chang, H.M., et al., *Pharmacology and Applications of Chinese Materia Medica*, Vol. 1. World Scientific Pub. 1986.

36. Vanderhoek, J., et al., "Inhibition of fatty acid lipoxygenases by onion and garlic oils: Evidence for the mechanism by which these oils inhibit platelet aggregation," *Biochem Pharmac*, 29:3169–73, 1980.

37. Dorsch, W. and Weber, J., "Prevention of allergen-induced bronchial constriction in sensitized guinea pigs by crude alcohol onion extract," *Agents and Actions*, 14:626–30, 1984.

38. Weerbach, Melvyn, M.D., *Healing Through Nutrition*, New York, Harper Collins Publishers, Inc. 1993, p. 35.

39. Middleton, E. and Drzewieki, G., "Naturally occurring flavonoids and human basophil histamine release," *Int. Arch. Allergy Appl Immunol*, 77:155–7, 1985; Amella M., Bronner, Briancon F., et al. "Inhibition of mast cell histamine release by flavonoids and bioflavonoids," *Planta Medica* 51:16–20, 1985.

40. Whitaker, Julian, M.D., *Dr. Whitaker's Guide To Natural Healing*, Rocklin, CA, Prima Publishing, 1994, p. 168.

41. Werbach, Melvyn, M.D., and Murray, Michael T., N.D., *Botanical Influences on Illness*, Tarzana, CA, Third Line Press, 1994, p. 320.

42. Subramanian, N., "Histamine degradation potential of ascorbic acid," *Agents and Actions* 8:484–7, 1978; Levine, M., "New concepts in the biology and biochemistry of ascorbic acid," *New England Journal of Medicine* 314:892–902, 1986.

43. Costarella, Linda, N.D., "Naturopathic Specific Condition Review: Asthma," In: *The Protocol Journal of Botanical Medicine*, Volume 1, Number 2, Autumn 1995, p. 102.

44. Gamble, Anne, "Alternative Medical Approaches to the Treatment of Asthma," *Alternative & Complementary Therapies,* Jan./Feb. 1995; pp. 61,63.

45. Willard, p. 117.

46. Hoffmann, David, *Therapeutic Herbalism,* A Correspondence Course in Phytotherapy. Chapter 2, p. 76.

47. Lih-Brody L., et al., "Increased oxidative stress and decreased antioxidant defenses in mucosa of inflammatory bowel disease, *Dig Dis Sci,* 41:2078–86, 1996.

48. Nielsen, O.H., et. al., "Involvement of oxygen free radicals in the pathogenesis of chronic inflammatory bowel disease," *Klin Wochenschr,* 69:995–1000, 1991.

49. Safayhi, H., et al., "Boswellic Acids: Novel, Specific, Nonredox Inhibitors of 5-lipoxygenase," *J Pharmacol Exp Thera,* 261(3): 203–7, June, 1992.

50. Zucker, Martin, "Ancient Indian Medical Herb Proving Itself a Winner for Modern Day Arthritis Sufferers," *Townsend Letter for Doctors,* Aug./Sept., p. 874, 1993.

51. Sodhi, Virender, M.D., N.D., *Ayurvedic Materia Medica: Inflammatory Diseases,* in Offical Proceedings of the Southwest Conference on Botanical Medicine, March 28–29, 1998 Tempe, Arizona, pp. 96–97.

52. Ibid.

53. van Loon, pg. 472–480.

54. Kasahara, Y., Kikino, H., et al., "Anti-inflammatory actions of ephedrines in acute inflammations," *Planta Medica,* 54:325–331, 1985.

55. Srivastava, K.D., and Mustafa, T., "Ginger *(Zingiber officinale)* in rheumatism and musculoskeletal disorders," *Med Hypotheses* (England), December, 39 (4), pp. 342–348, 1992.
Srivastava, K.D., and Mustafa, T., "Ginger (Zinger officinale) in migraine headache," *J Ethnopharmacol,* 29 (3):267–273, 1990.

56. Thurmon, F.M., "The treatment of psoriasis with a sarsaparilla compound," *New England Journal of Medicine,* 227:128–33, 1942.

137

57. Werbach, Melvyn R., M.D. and Murray, Michael T., N.D., *Botanical Influences on Illness*, Third Line Press: Tarzana, CA, 1994, pp. 216–217.
58. Bingham, R., et al., pp. 45–50.
59. Lamb, Bruce F., *Wizard of the Upper Amazon, The Story of Manuel Cordova-Rios*, Boston: Houghton-Mifflin Co., 1974, p. 199.

Resources

Blessed Herbs
Martha and Michael Volchok
109 Barre Plains Road
Oakham, MA 01068
Voice: 800–489–4372 / 508–882–3839
Fax: 508–882–3755

Frontier Cooperative Herbs
P.O. Box 299
Norway, IA 52318
Voice: 800–669–3275

Gaia Herbs
62 Old Littleton Road
Harvard, MA 01451
Voice: 800–831–7780 / 508–456–3049
Fax: 508–456–9154

Island Herbs
Ryan Drum
P.O. Box 25
Waldron Island, WA 98927–0025
Voice: 206–739–4035

Materia Medica
Tony Carter
4840 Pan American Freeway N.E., Suite A
Albuquerque, NM 87109
Voice: 800–553–4165 / 505–855–7720
Fax: 505–855–7725

Pacific Botanicals
Mark and Margie Wheeler
4350 Fish Hatchery Road
Grants Pass, OR 97527
Voice: 503–479–7777

R-U-VED Inc.,
S. Sodhi, N.D.
2115 112th Ave., NE
Bellevue, WA 98004
Voice: 800–925–1371 / 425–637–1400
(Quality Ayurvedic herbal products)

The Herb Pharm
Ed Smith
P.O. Box 116
Williams, OR 97544
Voice: 503–846–6262

Tieraona's Herbals
Tieraona Low Dog, M.D.
4840 Pan American Freeway N.E., Suite A
Albuquerque, NM 87109
Voice: 800–553–4165 / 505–855–7720
Fax: 505–855–7725

140

Westport Scandinavia
Distributor of Nordic Naturals ProOmega (70 percent Omega 3)
3040 Valencia Avenue, #2
Aptos, CA 95003
Voice: 800–662–2544 / 408–662–2852
Fax: 408–662–0382

Wise Woman Herbals, Inc.,
Sharon Tilgner, N.D.
P.O. Box 279
Creswell, OR 97426
Voice: 800–532–5219/541–895–5174

Index